SERVET

UPDATE

MAIN

ENDOCRINE DISORDERS

of the adrenal and thyroid axes

IN DOGS AND CATS

Víctor Castillo

SERVET

For this English edition:

Servet Update. *Main endocrine disorders of the adrenal and thyroid axes in dogs and cats*

Plaza Antonio Beltrán Martínez n° 1, planta 8 - letra I
(Centro empresarial El Trovador)
50002 Zaragoza - Spain

First printing: February 2018

This book has been published originally in Spanish under the title:
Servet Update. *Principales endocrinopatías de los ejes adrenal y tiroideo en perros y gatos*

ISBN Spanish edition: 978-84-17225-14-8

Translation:
Novalins

ISBN: 978-84-17225-38-4
D.L.: Z 105-2018

Design, layout and printing:
Servet editorial - Grupo Asís Biomedia, S.L.
www.grupoasis.com
info@grupoasis.com

Servet is the publishing house of Grupo Asís

Warning:

Veterinary science is constantly evolving, as are pharmacology and the other sciences. Inevitably, it is therefore the responsibility of the veterinary surgeon to determine and verify the dosage, the method of administration, the duration of treatment and any possible contraindications to the treatments given to each individual patient, based on his or her professional experience. Neither the publisher nor the author can be held liable for any damage or harm caused to people, animals or properties resulting from the correct or incorrect application of the information contained in this book.

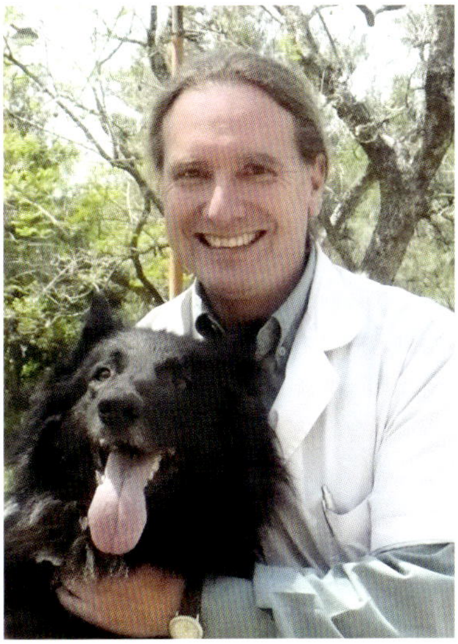

THE AUTHOR

Víctor Castillo

PhD, Specialist in Endocrinology

Víctor Castillo received his PhD in veterinary medicine from the University of Buenos Aires (UBA) in 2001. In 2003, he was awarded the title of Specialist in Endocrinology by the Argentine Society of Endocrinology and Metabolism, of which he has been a member since 1989. He is currently head for the veterinary area within the society's Advanced Course in Medical Endocrinology. He is assistant professor in the Department of Small Animal Clinical Medicine at the UBA. In addition to teaching endocrinology within the undergraduate curriculum, he is also head of the Endocrinology Unit at the UBA Veterinary Teaching Hospital and coordinates the internship programme in endocrinology at the UBA. The primary focus of his research is veterinary endocrinology, including thyroid and bone pathologies. Currently, his research centres on Cushing's syndrome. He is a director of research projects and doctoral and master's theses, and a tutor of interns and students in veterinary endocrinology. He also teaches several postgraduate specialisation courses, as well as graduate, master's, and doctoral programmes, both nationally and internationally. He has participated in many scientific events (congresses, conferences, courses), in the fields of both veterinary and human medicine. Within the field of veterinary endocrinology, he has published numerous scientific articles and spoken at many congresses. He is a reviewer of scientific articles for several international journals and is a member of several editorial committees.

PREFACE

Diseases of the endocrine system have always posed a diagnostic and therapeutic challenge, since the same disease can manifest clinically in a variety of ways.

Disorders of the adrenal and thyroid axes are among the most common within the field of veterinary endocrinology. Owing to the slow and progressive course of endocrine diseases, their diagnosis is often established late. Many professionals wait for the onset of the classic signs of these diseases. However, while often seen in photographs, these signs are rarely observed during consultation. Experience has also shown that in many countries and localities, diagnosis is complicated by a lack of availability of the most commonly described methodologies. The failure to consider other diagnostic methods that could provide the same results is a source of significant frustration for clinicians. Although it is important to establish widely agreed upon diagnostic criteria, it is no less important to be able to establish a diagnosis using alternative methods that are simple, accessible, and adapted to regional realities. For example, it is easier to perform a urinary cortisol/creatinine test than an 8-hour dexamethasone inhibition test in low-income areas or in situations in which owners do not wish to leave their pet in the clinic for a long period of time.

This same criterion also applies to treatment; not all owners in all countries can purchase certain drugs, but they may be able to afford alternatives that are effective in a large percentage of cases.

This book is designed as a tool and a guide for the veterinary clinician to aid the diagnosis of common diseases of the endocrine system, such as Cushing's syndrome and hypothyroidism, as well as other less frequent disorders such as adrenal insufficiency and hyperthyroidism. Different approaches are presented to establish a diagnosis and to select and administer the appropriate treatment, which should be available and accessible within the veterinary clinician's place of work.

Víctor Castillo

TABLE OF CONTENTS

CUSHING'S SYNDROME

REGULATORY CHARACTERISTICS OF THE HYPOTHALAMIC–PITUITARY–ADRENAL (HPA) AXIS

The HPA axis should be considered as a functional unit with interrelated components (Fig. 1). From the paraventricular nucleus of the hypothalamus, corticotropin-releasing factor (CRF) and antidiuretic hormone or vasopressin (ADH/VAP), which act on the pars distalis (adenohypophysis or anterior lobe), are released onto a group of cells called corticotropes. These cells in turn synthesise a macromolecule (proopiomelanocortin, POMC) that is broken down into groups of amino acids; one such group is the 39-amino-acid adrenocorticotropic hormone (ACTH). Other adrenal axis stimulators include adrenaline, inflammatory cytokines, oestradiol, and angiotensin. [1,2] Negative regulation (inhibition of synthesis) of corticotropic cells is mainly mediated by cortisol, but also by somatostatin and dopamine. [3] This is of therapeutic importance. CRF also acts on the corticotropic cells of the pars intermedia, which is innervated but not irrigated, inducing POMC synthesis via an enzymatic step. In this case, the first 14 amino acids of ACTH are cleaved to produce melanocyte-stimulating hormone (α-MSH). The pars intermedia is regulated by dopamine. When dopamine levels increase, ACTH is processed, increasing levels of α-MSH. A decrease in dopamine levels has the opposite effect, increasing ACTH levels. [4] The decrease in dopamine levels that accompanies ageing results in increased activity of the adrenal axis. [5]

The following are specific traits of the adrenal axis that help to explain Cushing's syndrome:

- Sexual dimorphism, in terms of both corticotrope morphology and adrenal axis function. In the female, the size of corticotropic cells changes with the oestrous cycle. This sexual dimorphism is also evident when the adrenal gland (AG) is stimulated or the adrenal axis is inhibited (females show an enhanced response to stimulation and a longer period of inhibition, respectively). [6]
- Dissociation between AG and ACTH; because the AG has secretory autonomy, its sensitivity varies throughout the day, and it is stimulated by other agents (cytokines, luteinising hormone [LH], innervation of the autonomic nervous system, various peptides). [7]

The left AG is located near the abdominal aorta and is shaped like an eight, while the right gland is located near the caudal vena cava and is shaped like an inverted triangle (Fig. 1). The latter is often difficult to visualise in ultrasound studies.

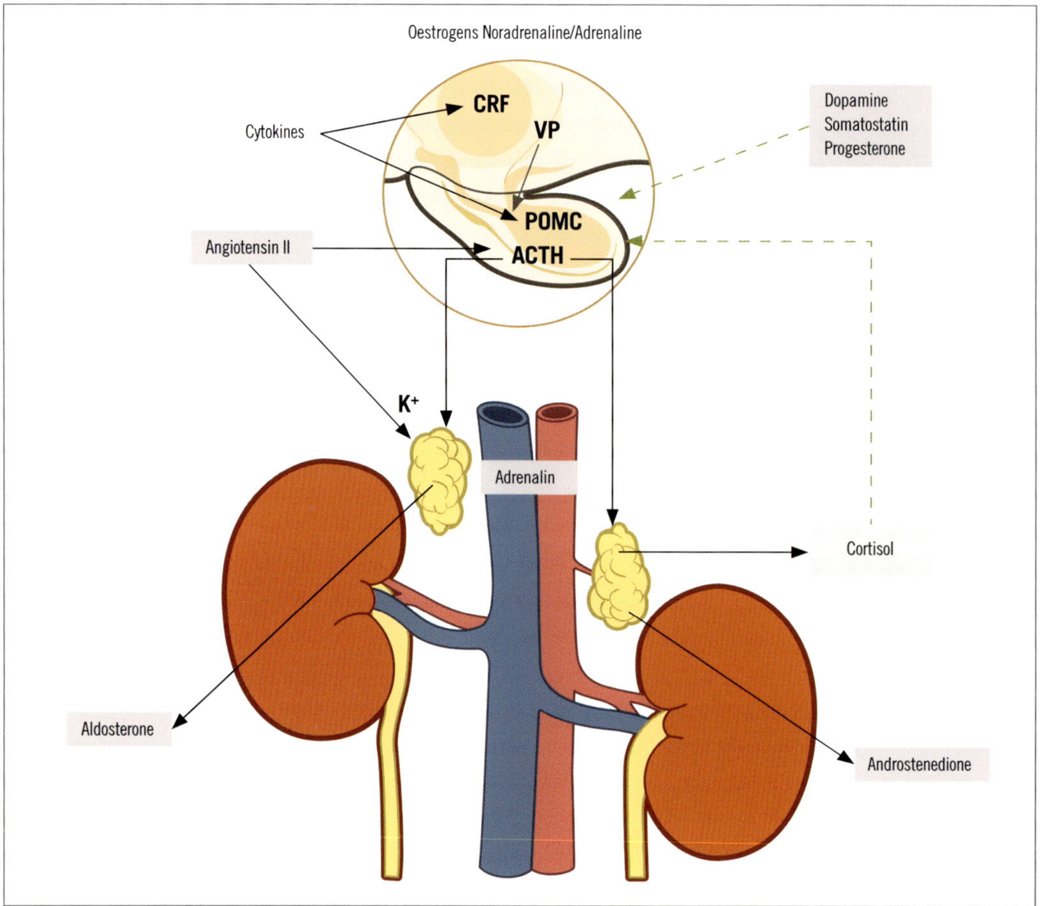

Figure 1. Regulation of the HPA axis and location of the AGs. Activators (solid arrows) and inhibitors (dashed arrows). The AGs are located near the abdominal aorta and the vena cava.

Each AG consists of two parts: the cortex and medulla (Fig. 1). The cortex is divided into three histologically and functionally distinct parts:

- Glomerular or arcuate zone: synthesises mineralocorticoids (aldosterone).
- Fascicular zone: synthesises glucocorticoids (cortisol).
- Reticular zone: synthesises androgens (androstenedione).

The medulla mainly synthesises adrenaline, and is innervated by the autonomic nervous system.

ACTH receptors are found in the membrane of adrenal cortex cells and, when stimulated, trigger the synthesis of steroid hormones, mainly cortisol and androstenedione. This process is mediated by the entry of cholesterol and a subsequent complex process involving a series of enzymatic steps. Once the hormones have been synthesised, they are released into the peripheral circulation. In the glomerular zone, the action of ACTH is of little relevance, whereas potassium (increases) and angiotensin II are important to induce aldosterone synthesis. [1]

AETIOLOGY

Cushing's syndrome (CS) is defined as an increase in the concentration of cortisol, due either to increased stimulation of its synthesis or to increased secretion of ACTH or LH resulting from autonomous or independent production in the fascicular area.

CS can be classified as ACTH-dependent or ACTH-independent. [8] Knowledge of this classification and the underlying causes facilitates the diagnosis and treatment:

ACTH-dependent (ACTHd-CS)

Accounts for 80–83 % of cases. Two variants are described:

- Pituitary-dependent (PDCS): hypersecretion of ACTH by corticotropic cells. Can be due to the presence of an ACTH-producing pituitary adenoma (corticotropinoma) as the primary cause (Fig. 2), or to disinhibition of corticotropic cells caused by a decrease in dopamine, a situation seen in senior dogs.
- Ectopic ACTH secretion: known as ectopic ACTH syndrome. This is associated with carcinoid tumours and neuroendocrine tumours or apudomas. To date, three cases have been reported in dogs. [9,10,11]

ACTH-independent (ACTHi-CS)

Cortisol secretion is independent of ACTH stimulation. Accounts for 17–20 % of cases. Possible causes include:

- Adrenal tumour (AT): 95 % of ACTHi cases. Presence of an AG adenoma (40 %) or carcinoma (55 %) (Fig. 2).
- Macronodular adrenal hyperplasia (MAH): formation of nodules (unilateral or bilateral) in the AG (often confused with adenomas), caused by an exaggerated reaction to normal stimulation of ACTH, gastric inhibitory peptide (GIP), or the autonomous nervous system.
- Illegitimate receptors in the AG: these are receptors for other hormones or peptides, such as LH or GIP, that are expressed in the AG and induce cortisol synthesis. Both have been reported in dogs and cause bilateral AG hyperplasia. [13.14]

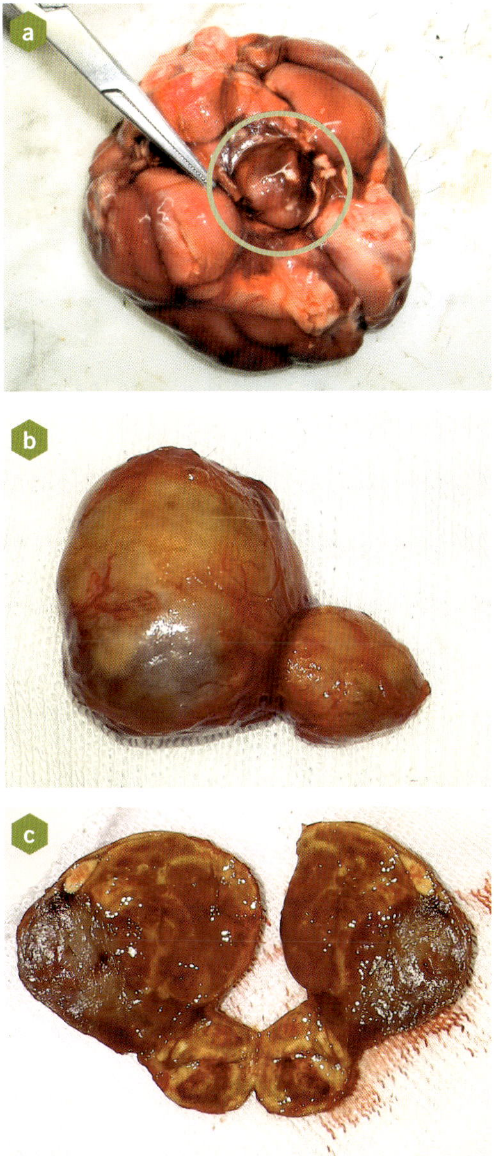

Figure 2. (a) Macroadenoma (corticotropinoma). (b and c) Adrenal cortex carcinomas in the fascicular area.

PREDISPOSITION BY SPECIES, BREED, AND SEX

This disease affects humans, dogs, cats, horses, ferrets, and monkeys. It can occur in young dogs (2–4 years of age). Although it can be diagnosed between 13 and 16 years of age, it is more frequently diagnosed in animals of 7–9 years of age. [1] In cats, ferrets, and horses it is diagnosed in adults. Its prevalence and incidence is high in dogs. [1] It is very rare in cats, whereas in horses the only form described is that originating in the pars intermedia (equine pituitary pars intermedia dysfunction [PPID]). In ferrets, in contrast to dogs, cats, and humans, the main cause is an AT (80 %). [14]

Breed predisposition can vary depending on the country, the preferences of the population for certain breeds, and the prevalence of mixed-breed dogs. The Poodle is highly predisposed to this disease, which also commonly affects the Boxer, Dachshund, Beagle, Labrador, Golden Retriever, Miniature Schnauzer, and Pitbull. According to a study carried out in Buenos Aires (Argentina) that examined 500 cases of CS over 10 years, 30 % of the cases involved mixed-breed dogs, with the remaining 70 % distributed among different breeds (Table 1).

CS is more prevalent in females than in males (3:1 ratio). This difference is observed in all affected species, and applies to the two main aetiologies (PDCS and AT-CS). [1,15]

Table 1. Percentage distribution of CS by breed in 500 cases (2006–2016).

Dogs with CS (ACTHd and ACTHi)	Distribution (%)
Mixed-breed	27
Poodle	14
Beagle	10
Miniature Schnauzer	9
Dachshund	7
Boxer	5
Golden Retriever	4
Labrador Retriever	3
Pitbull	2
Other breeds *	19

* German Shepherd, Fox Terrier, American Staffordshire Terrier, Dalmatian, French Bulldog, Bichon Frisé, Breton Spaniel, Yorkshire Terrier, Shar Pei, Siberian Husky, Rhodesian Ridgeback, Chow Chow.

CLINICAL SIGNS AND ASSOCIATED COMORBIDITIES

The clinical presentation of CS is, in general, the same in ACTH-dependent and -independent cases. It should be borne in mind that when an animal is diagnosed with an AT, diagnosis is late from the oncological point of view, since the tumour will already have reached a considerable size. Cortisol secretion is directly related to the size of the tumour, which grows slowly but progressively. Clinical signs become apparent when the adrenal tumour is ≥1 cm, and appear more rapidly in cases of PDCS.

CS can present subclinically or can be oligosymptomatic (with only mild clinical expression), with a variable duration (2–5 years). [8,16] During this period, the clinical signs suggestive of this disorder are a sustained increase in weight perceived by the owner, with changes in the appearance of the abdomen, and the presence of recurrent pyoderma. Females may be in heat or anoestrous for some time. This allows us to estimate the course of the disease, since the gonadal axis is quickly inhibited by the increase in cortisol levels. [15] The most significant changes are revealed by blood chemistry profiles, which show an increase in alkaline phosphatase (ALP), fasting hyperglycaemia (glucose values of 100–130 mg/dl, or even diabetes mellitus), and hypercholesterolaemia. Breeds such as the Miniature Schnauzer, Beagle, Dachshund, and the Siberian Husky (Fig. 3) usually develop the subclinical form of this disease.

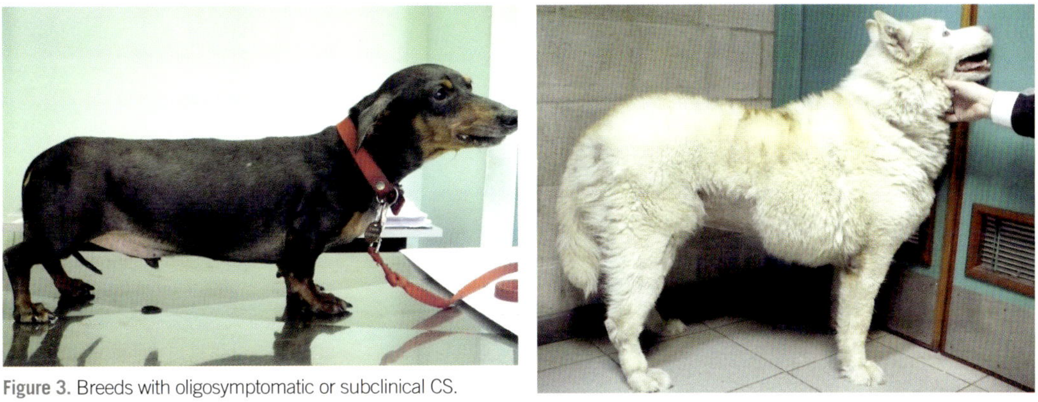

Figure 3. Breeds with oligosymptomatic or subclinical CS.

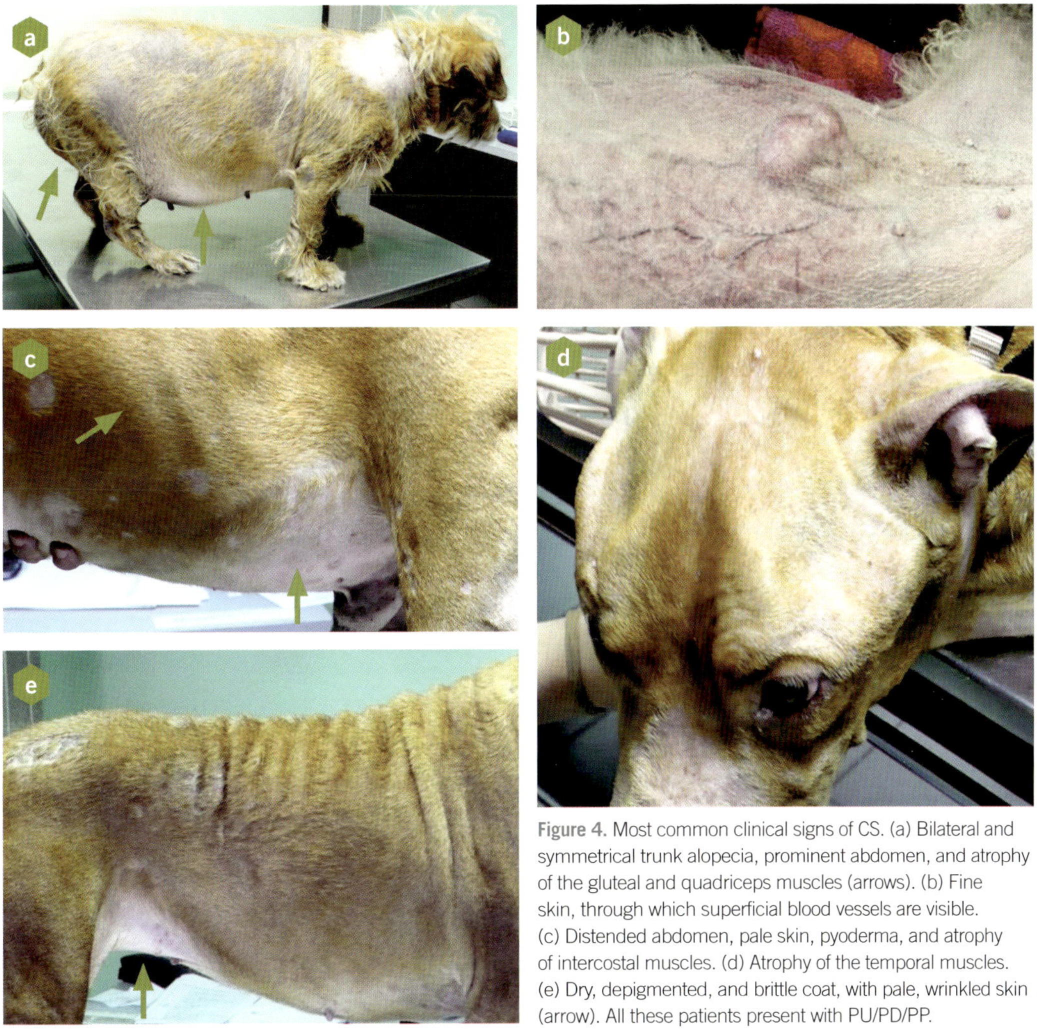

Figure 4. Most common clinical signs of CS. (a) Bilateral and symmetrical trunk alopecia, prominent abdomen, and atrophy of the gluteal and quadriceps muscles (arrows). (b) Fine skin, through which superficial blood vessels are visible. (c) Distended abdomen, pale skin, pyoderma, and atrophy of intercostal muscles. (d) Atrophy of the temporal muscles. (e) Dry, depigmented, and brittle coat, with pale, wrinkled skin (arrow). All these patients present with PU/PD/PP.

Table 2. Common clinical signs in CS.

Clinical signs	Frequency
PU/PD	++++ (not in cats, except those with diabetes)
PP	+++
Dermatological signs:	
▶ Hair:	
▶ Hair loss/alopecia	+++ (rare in cats, absent in horses)
▶ Dry, bristly hair	+++
▶ Depigmentation	+
▶ Excessive hair growth	Only in horses
▶ Skin:	
▶ Loses elasticity and becomes coarse	++++
▶ Colour changes	++ (paleness in Boxers and Pitbulls)
▶ Calcinosis cutis	+
Prominent (bulging) abdomen	++++
Muscular atrophy (gluteal, quadriceps, temporal/ intercostal, and lumbar muscles)	++ (the gluteal and quadriceps muscles are initially affected, followed by the temporal and intercostal muscles, and finally the lumbar muscles in very advanced stages)
Anoestrous/absence of libido	+++ (early sign of onset of CS)
Oedematous vulva	Only in ferrets
Exercise intolerance	+++ (associated with muscular atrophy)
Tachypnoea (severe wheezing) or shortness of breath	+ (associated with muscle atrophy or signs of hypertension or thromboembolism in CS)

The clinical form (Fig. 4) is the most common. [1,8] Clinical signs are characteristic of the disease (Table 2), and include polyuria, polydipsia, polyphagia (PU/PD/PP), a distended abdomen (not usually seen in Boxers or Dachshunds), and thin and inelastic skin. The owner will notice that the animal develops exercise intolerance due to muscle atrophy, which usually affects the gluteus, quadriceps, and intercostal muscles. Atrophy of the temporal and lumbar muscles is observed in advanced stages of the disease. Hair loss varies depending on the breed and coat type. It should therefore be borne in mind that the clinical signs affecting the haircoat and skin and the appearance of the abdomen may differ between breeds/mixed-breed dogs (Figs. 4 and 5). The presence of tachypnoea is cause to suspect severe arterial hypertension with or without pulmonary thromboembolism (Fig. 6).

Cats with CS are usually obese, and can also have associated diabetes mellitus (presenting complaint). Haircoats may undergo changes in structure (dryness), but without alopecia. As in humans, cats do not present with PU/PD unless they also have diabetes mellitus. Another frequent sign is lowered ears. Cats with an AT tend to lose weight. Acromegaly should be included in the differential diagnosis.

CS has several comorbidities (Table 3), which should be taken into account and treated, since some may lead to death (pulmonary thromboembolism, renal failure) or decrease life expectancy or quality of life (diabetes mellitus, dyslipidaemia, hypothyroidism). [8,17]

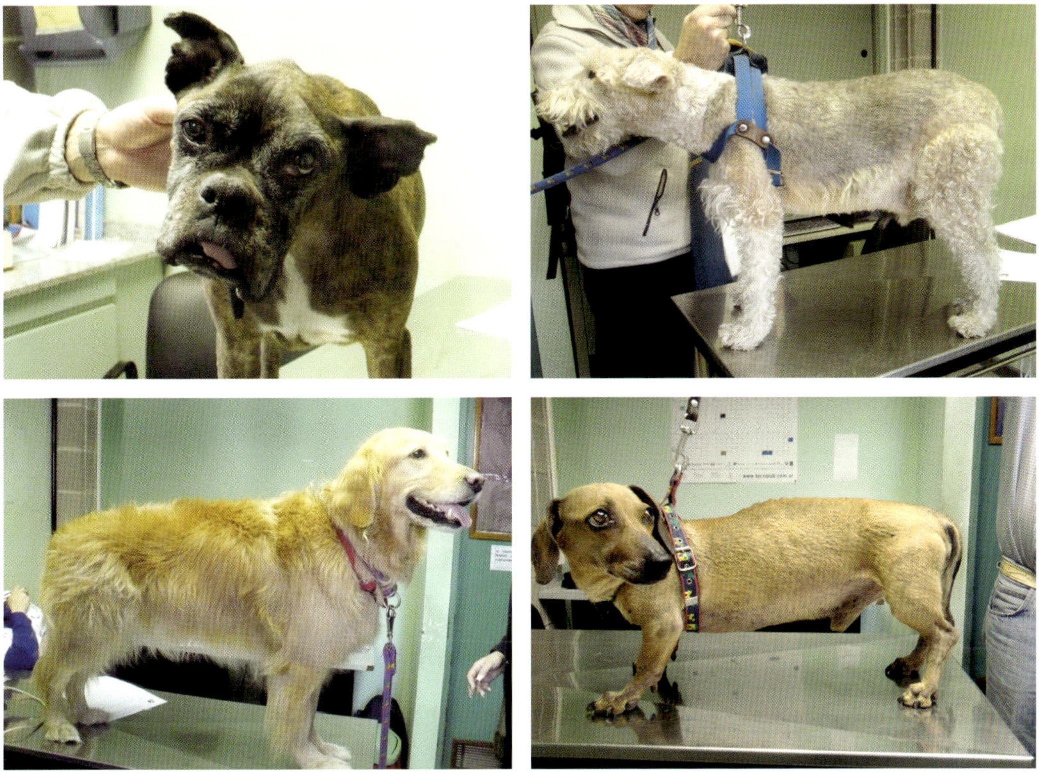

Figure 5. Different clinical manifestations of CS according to breed.

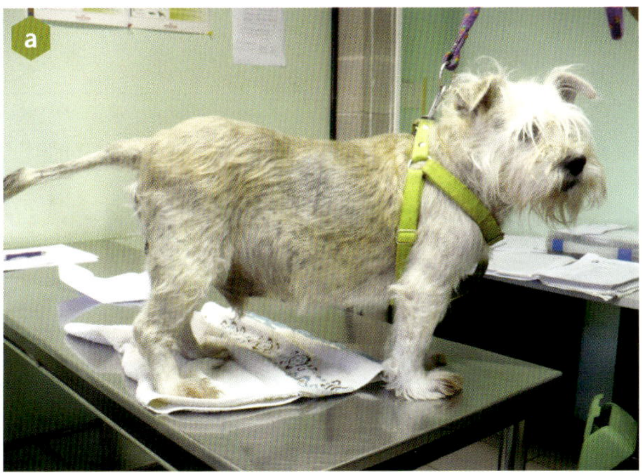

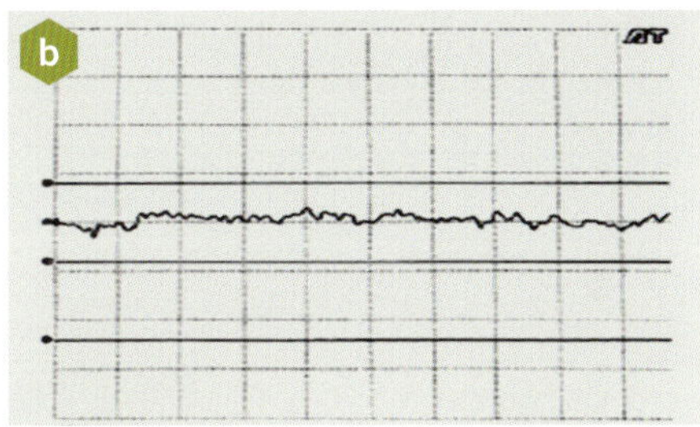

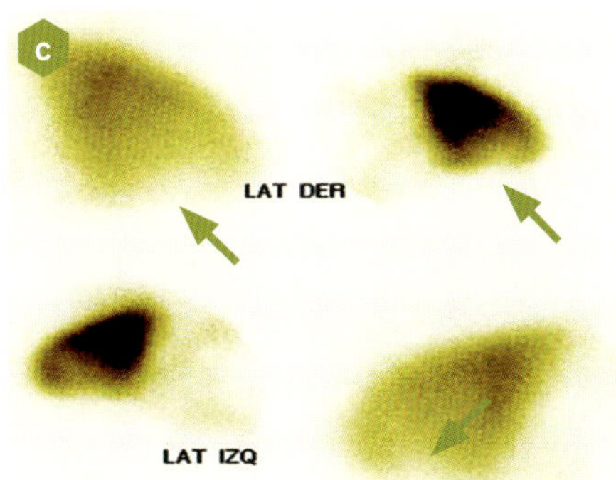

Figure 6. (a) Patient with typical signs of this disease, in addition to sudden-onset blindness, tachypnoea, and agitation at rest. (b) Electroretinography reveals blindness due to retinal injury ("flat" waves) and (c) scintigraphy reveals pulmonary thromboembolism (arrows). This dog has arterial hypertension and the MRI indicates the presence of a 6-mm pituitary tumour without involvement of the optic chiasm.

Table 3. Comorbidities resulting from or associated with CS (n = 350).

Comorbidities	Presentation (%)
Rapid-onset blindness	8
Hypertension (depending on whether systolic pressure is evaluated alone or together with diastolic pressure)	60–80
Nephropathy/renal failure	40–50
Hypercoagulation	25
Pulmonary embolism	5
Diabetes mellitus	12
Fasting glucose intolerance/fasting hyperglycaemia (100–150 mg/dl glucose)	30
Dyslipidaemia (hypercholesterolaemia, hypertriglyceridaemia)	80
Associated hypothyroidism	40
Neurological signs due to the compressive effect of the pituitary tumour or stroke due to rupture or necrosis of tumoural blood vessels	3
Vascular/haemodynamic signs due to invasion of the vena cava by the tumour of the right AG (hindlimb oedema, internal haemorrhage due to rupture of the vena cava or aortic artery)	2

Table 4. Laboratory test parameters (routine biochemistry) frequently altered in CS (diagnostically useful).

Analyte	Frequency
Liver enzymes:	
▸ ALP	++++
▸ ALT (GPT)	+++
▸ AST (GOT)	+
Metabolism:	
▸ Glucose	++ (>100 mg/dl fasting)
▸ Total cholesterol	+++
▸ Triglycerides	+++
Ionogram:	
▸ Na^+ and K^+	+ (only in AT)
Urine:	
▸ Urinary density	+++
▸ UPC (protein/creatinine ratio)	++

DIAGNOSIS

Routine chemistry profiles can help guide diagnosis. Table 4 summarises the most important parameters to be taken into account, given the frequency with which they are altered.

Definitive diagnosis of CS and its origin is based on endocrine biochemistry, which requires the use of dynamic tests. The indication and choice of these tests depends very much on their availability in a given region or country, on the availability of certain drugs used for diagnostic purposes, and on local idiosyncrasies (certain owners may be averse to long-term or invasive tests, may have economic constraints, or may not wish to hospitalise their pet for analyses, etc.). Therefore, it is recommended to consult a local clinician regarding the diagnostic test best adapted to the particular situation in a given region or country. No diagnostic test has a sensitivity of 100 % (usual range, 75–83 %). Therefore, in the case of a negative test result, the disease should not be ruled out, nor should

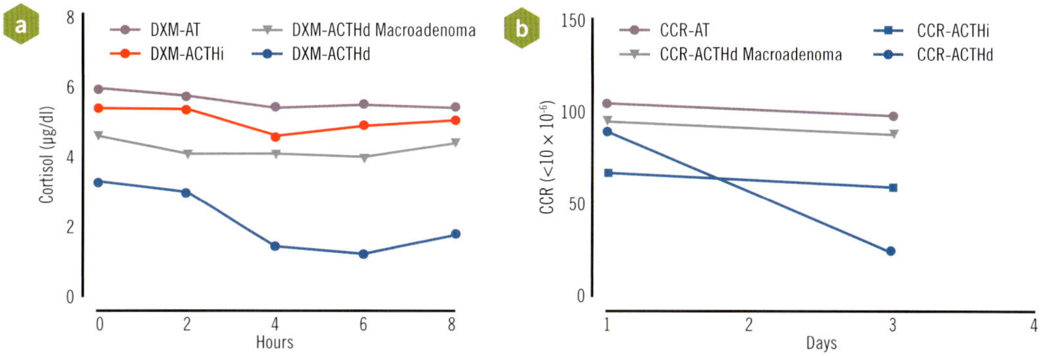

Figure 7. (a) Inhibition with a low IV dose of DXM and (b) inhibition with a high dose of DXM in urine (CCR-DXM). Note the expected inhibitory response (blue) in the case of pituitary tumour (PD-CS). Three responses in which no inhibition is observed are also shown (in two cases due to causes other than the presence of an AT).

the origin be assumed; a second test or an imaging study are necessary to corroborate the diagnosis. The most commonly used tests are briefly described below. Table 5 lists the pros and cons of the different diagnostic tests.

- Measurement of plasma ACTH: high values or those close to the upper limit indicate ACTHd-CS, while values close to or below the lower limit are suggestive of ACTHi-CS and indicate the need for imaging analyses to determine the presence of an AT. The limiting factor is the management of sample collection and transport, since ACTH is rapidly inactivated. Blood is collected in pre-refrigerated plastic tubes containing an anticoagulant (EDTA) and, if possible, aprotinin (delays ACTH degradation). The sample is immediately centrifuged and frozen at 30 °C until processing (it should be frozen for transport to the laboratory if collected in the veterinary clinic). ACTH concentrations should be analysed in parallel with those of cortisol (plasma or urinary).
- Urinary cortisol/creatinine ratio (CCR) (baseline and after inhibition with oral dexamethasone [DXM]): [8,19] samples of the second urine passed in the morning, night urine, and the first urine passed the following morning should be collected in the same container (intermediate samples may also be collected). From this sample the pre-dexamethasone (DXM1) CCR value is obtained. Elevated values are indicative of CS. Immediately after this first sampling, oral DXM (0.1 mg/kg) is administered every 8 hours. The next day, the first urine of the morning is collected and the post-dexamethasone CCR value (DXM2) is compared with DXM1. A DXM2 value ≤50 % of the DXM1 value is indicative of PD-CS. For samples to be homogeneous, the owner should retain 1 ml of urine from each collection.
- Inhibition with low-dose DXM (0.01 mg/kg/IV): should be evaluated 2, 4, 6, and 8 hours after DXM administration. The absence of inhibition at 2 hours is diagnostic of CS. Inhibition at 4 or 6 hours indicates PD-CS.

It should be noted that both DXM inhibition tests (urine and IV) have a sensitivity of 75–80 %, [18] and therefore the absence of inhibition does not indicate that the syndrome is of adrenal origin (Table 5 and Fig. 7). Therefore, the results obtained should be confirmed with imaging studies of the AG and pituitary.

Table 5. Diagnostic tests frequently used in CS.

Diagnostic tests	Sensitivity (%)	False positives (do not have CS or are considered positive if DXM causes inhibition)	False negatives (have CS or DXM does not cause inhibition)
CS diagnosis only: ▸ Stimulation with ACTH ▸ CCR	 80 80	Acute or chronic stress, diabetes mellitus or insipida, pheochromocytoma, obesity	Illegitimate receptor, adrenal carcinoma (ACTH stimulation), incipient CS (both)
CS diagnosis and origin: ▸ Inhibition with low-dose DXM (IV) ▸ Inhibition with high-dose DXM in urine	 75–80 80	Diagnostic error (the animal does not have CS), nonfunctioning adrenal cortex tumour, or adrenal medulla tumour	Pituitary macroadenoma, origin in pars intermedia, management stress (IV), CS due to illegitimate receptors or ectopic ACTH syndrome, diabetes mellitus, previous corticotherapy
Differential diagnosis of ACTHd-CS and ACTHi-CS: ▸ Measurement of plasma ACTH (does not discriminate between pituitary ACTH and ectopic ACTH, although in these cases the concentrations are usually higher)	90 (together with some previous test)	Management stress (acute), inadequate laboratory tests	Inadequate sample handling (inactivation in the absence of an AT), previous administration of exogenous corticosteroids (inhibition in the absence of an AT), inadequate laboratory tests

Diagnostic imaging

Essential for diagnostic confirmation and to determine tumour location and size, the involvement of neighbouring structures, therapeutic approach, and surgical risk. The most commonly used methods are described below.

Ultrasound

This is the imaging method of choice. Moreover, it is accessible to clinicians in most countries. Ultrasound allows visualisation of both AGs. An AG width >7 mm with a hypoechoic appearance is considered indicative of adrenal hyperplasia (Fig. 8). However, the absence of changes in echogenicity and/or size does not rule out the presence of a functional abnormality. Bilateral hyperplasia is not always indicative of PD-CS, and may be due to other causes. Ultrasound is mainly used for the diagnosis of AT. A Doppler study reveals the presence of a tumoural embolus in the vena cava in cases of right adrenal gland tumour. [20]

Computed tomography (CT) and magnetic resonance imaging (MRI)

These methods have a high level of diagnostic sensitivity. However, CT is preferable in cases of AT (Fig. 9), since it provides better resolution in the abdomen than MRI, although its sensitivity in evaluating the sellar region (sella turcica) is lower, except in the case of 3-D CT. [21]

MRI is the method of choice for studying the pituitary gland, [15] and determining the size of the tumour and its projection (Fig. 10); coronal, sagittal, and axial sections may be requested. Depending on the image obtained, pituitary tumours can be classified as macroadenomas with extrasellar extension (>5 mm, surpassing the borders of the sella turcica) or

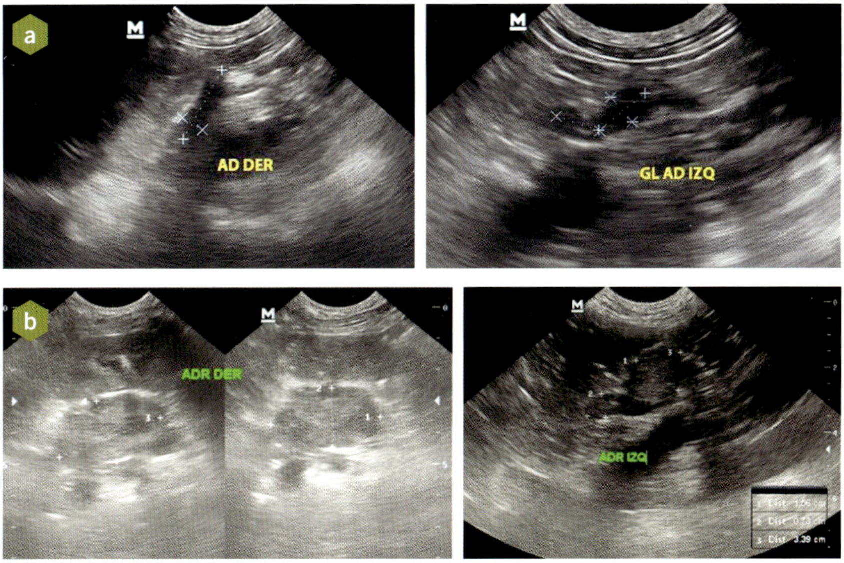

Figure 8. Ultrasonography of (a) hyperplastic and (b) tumoural AGs.

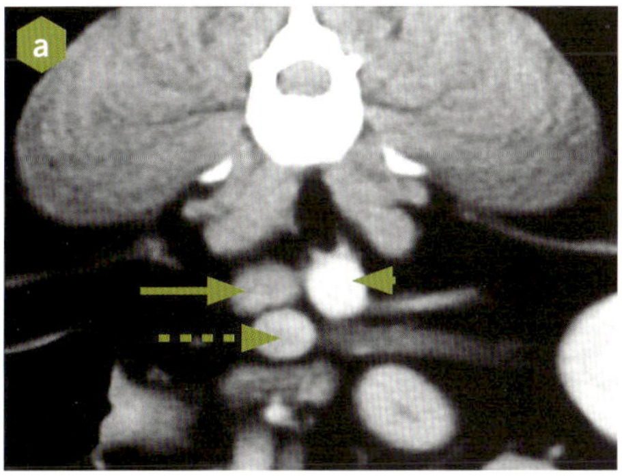

Figure 9. CT. (a) Circumscribed AT (solid arrow) that does not contact the vena cava (dashed arrow) or the abdominal aorta (tip of arrow). (b and c) Large ATs (adrenal cortex carcinomas) (solid arrow) that affect the blood vessels (dashed arrow).

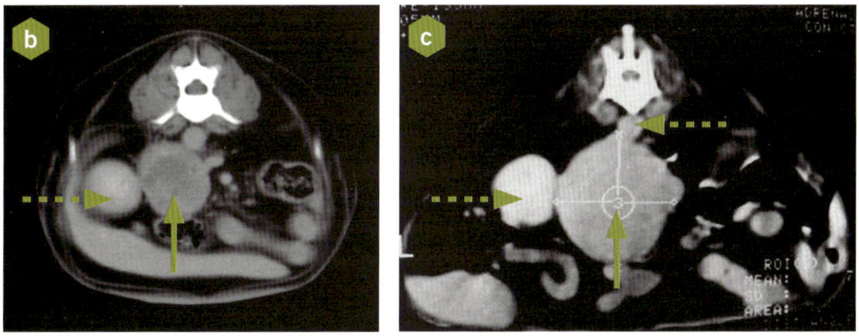

as microadenomas with intrasellar extension (2–5 mm).[15] The absence of pituitary disease in MRI images does not rule out the presence of a microadenoma. Therefore, these images should be interpreted together with the results of laboratory diagnostic tests, and the possibility of ectopic ACTH syndrome or illegitimate LH or GIP receptors in the AG.

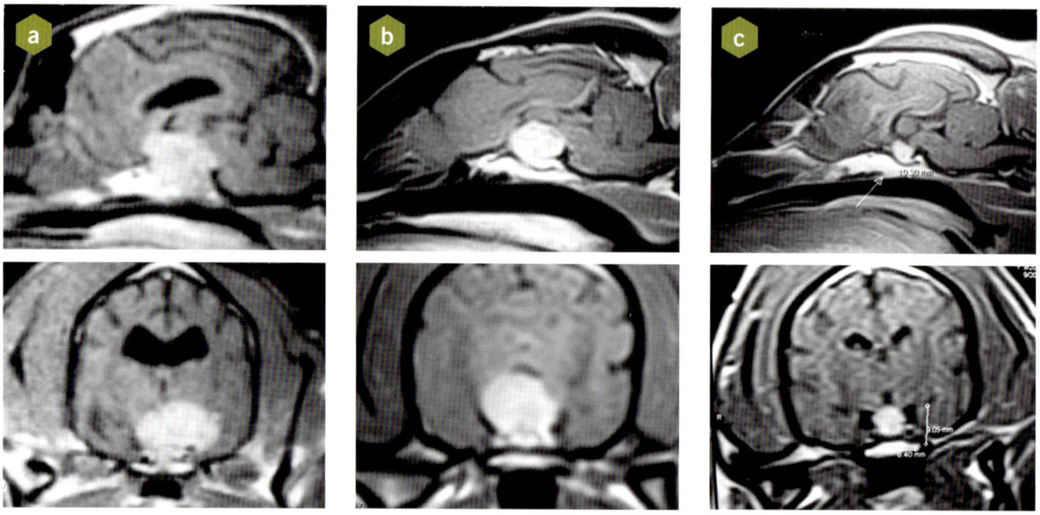

Figure 10. MRI (sagittal and coronal views). (a) Aggressive and invasive pituitary tumour, the location of which causes tilting of the patient's head. (b) Aggressive tumour that exerts a mass effect. (c) Delimited and nonaggressive pituitary tumour of 7 mm that responds well to drug treatment.

TREATMENT

Treatment depends on the origin of the syndrome. No treatment is 100 % effective (most are 75–80 % effective). [1,22,23] This is due to relapse (for both pituitary and adrenal tumours), resistance, habituation, or intolerance to drug treatments, or adverse effects. CS comorbidities, particularly arterial hypertension, renal function disorders, and hyperglycaemia, should also be controlled. The most commonly used treatments for PD-CS and AT-CS are described below (Fig. 11).

PD-CS

Drug treatment or pituitary surgery.

Drug treatment can inhibit cortisol synthesis in the AG or inhibit ACTH synthesis and tumour growth by inducing apoptosis of neoplastic cells. The current approach is to combine two or more drugs.

Drugs that act on the AG (Table 6)

Trilostane is commonly administered [25] at a dose of 0.2–1.1 mg/kg/12 hours, [24] with ACTH stimulation at 15–20 days, which is repeated periodically every 15–20 days until the poststimulation cortisol concentration is ≤7 µg/dl (i.e. the gland is inhibited). A maintenance dose of 0.2 mg/kg/24 hours is then administered up until another ACTH stimulation test is performed at 20–30 days. If significant inhibition is observed, a weekly dose is administered. The disadvantage of this drug is its lack of availability in many countries; its cost, which is increased owing to the need for periodic follow-up treatment; and the lack of availability of synthetic ACTH (tetracosactrin), which is required for adequate therapeutic control.

Ketoconazole (KTZ) at a dose of 20–30 mg/kg/day in a single daily dose (starting with the lowest dose) is effective in 40 % of cases based on this author's experience, and does not have

Table 6. Treatments indicated in cases of PD-CS and AT-CS.

Treatment	PD-CS	AT-CS
Steroidogenesis inhibitors	KTZ, trilostane (risk of adrenal insufficiency)	Trilostane, mitotane, or KTZ * (inhibit the production of cortisol by the tumour or its metastases)
Antiapoptotics and inhibitors of POMC-ACTH synthesis (act at the pituitary gland)	AR 9-cis, Cbg, pergolide (horses), selegiline, pasireotide (SOM230), deslorelin ** (ferrets)	
Surgical treatment	Hypophysectomy	Tumour adrenalectomy

* Indicated when the tumour cannot be removed, either on the recommendation of a veterinary surgeon or because the owner does not consent, or in cases of metastasis in combination with chemotherapy.

** Inhibits the gonadal axis through its action as a GnRH agonist, decreases LH, and prevents AG stimulation.

the added risk of causing adrenal insufficiency. It is not recommended for use for more than 6 to 7 months, and can be re-administered if clinical signs reappear. [1,26]

The mean survival time with these drugs is 2 years. However, corticotropinomas can develop rapidly in response to the decreased inhibitory effect associated with the reduction in cortisol levels. [26,27]

Drugs that act on the pituitary (Table 6)

These are effective for the treatment of ACTH-secreting adenomas of <8 mm, but less so for larger tumours. This caveat also applies to pituitary surgery. [28]

Dopaminergic drugs increase dopamine levels, inhibiting ACTH and α-MSH secretion. These include selegiline and cabergoline (Cbg). [28,29] The latter is administered at a dose of 0.07–0.1 mg/kg/week, dividing the total weekly dose into 7 daily doses (0.125–2 mg total/day, depending on the patient's weight). Treatment should begin at the lowest dose, which is gradually increased according to the clinical response observed (normalisation of fluid and food intake, weight loss, etc.). Given the idiosyncratic sensitivity of miniature Schnauzers to Cbg, treatment of these dogs should begin at half the aforementioned dose. This also applies to cats with CS. The response to treatment with this drug depends on whether or not the corticotropinoma expresses short D2 dopamine receptors. It is effective in 40 % of cases, with an initial response observed in 60 % of treated dogs. Resistance to Cbg, if initially effective, occurs between 2 and 4 months after beginning treatment. If no clinical response is observed within 2 months of starting Cbg treatment, treatment with a different drug is recommended. However, Cbg can be administered for years without any problem in animals that show a good response. Concomitant levothyroxine treatment is advisable to prevent inhibition of the thyroid axis.

Inhibitors of ACTH synthesis and inducers of tumour apoptosis

This group includes retinoic acid (RA) in the form of isotretinoin 9-cis (2°mg/kg/day PO), and pasireotide or SOM230. [22,28,30,31]

RA is effective in the control and remission of CS in 80 % of treated dogs. The desired effect (clinical signs, decrease in CCR) is generally not observed for 2 to 3 months. If this occurs, treatment is continued for 6 to 8 months while monitoring the liver profile. [26] Treatment is frequently associated with an increase in triglyceride levels, which causes hypothyroidism. As such, concomitant administration of levothyroxine is advisable. On discontinuation of treatment, animals that have responded well do not relapse within the following 2 years. This drug can be combined with Cbg, as both target common molecular signalling pathways and therefore enhance each other's effects.

Pasireotide or SOM230 is an analogue of somatostatin that inhibits tumour growth and ACTH synthesis. It should be administered (lyophilised form) at a dose of 0.04 µg/kg/12 hours (SC). A long-acting form can be administered at a dose of 4–6 mg/kg/month, but can be associated with hypotension and increased defecation frequency. No increase in blood glucose has been reported, in line with findings in humans. Both forms can be combined with Cbg.

For therapeutic control the CCR is monitored. This parameter should decrease relative to initial values. It should be measured every 3 months and, once stabilised at reference value levels, every 6 months. The mean survival time of a patient treated with Cbg and RA is 3 to 4 years. Death is due to natural causes or age-related diseases. Cortisol concentrations remain within normal ranges.

Pituitary surgery

This approach is not commonly used in veterinary medicine and requires highly trained personnel. The postoperative recurrence rate for pituitary surgery is 23 % [23] and it is not indicated in senior animals or those with macroadenoma.

Adrenal tumour (AT)

Adrenalectomy is indicated, although an attempt may be made to control cortisol secretion with trilostane or high doses of KTZ [1,25,32] prior to gland excision. These drugs only inhibit tumour growth in cases of carcinoma. Good pre-, intra-, and postoperative management is essential:

- Preoperative: control of blood pressure.
- Intraoperative: use of anticoagulants, control of blood pressure, and IV administration of hydrocortisone (300 mg/500 ml saline solution, administered by drip at 30 drops/minute).
- Postoperative: after tumour removal, the patient should remain hospitalised given the possibility of life-threatening complications such as haemorrhages, electrolyte imbalance, pulmonary thromboembolism, and hypertensive crisis. It is advisable to treat the patient with heparin or fibrinolytics for at least 5 to 7 days and to perform serial ionograms during the postoperative period. Hydrocortisone (0.51 mg/kg) should be administered for at least 2 to 3 months after surgery, beginning with one dose every 12 hours and subsequently decreasing to once per week, with continued ionogram monitoring. Once hydrocortisone treatment is discontinued, the recovery of adrenal function is evaluated by means of the ACTH test. Cortisol values of 13–15 µg/dl at 1 hour poststimulation are considered indicative of a satisfactory outcome. It is advisable to assess the adrenal region by thoracic radiography every 6 months to monitor for possible metastasis, which can occur between 4 months and 4 years after surgery (Fig. 11).

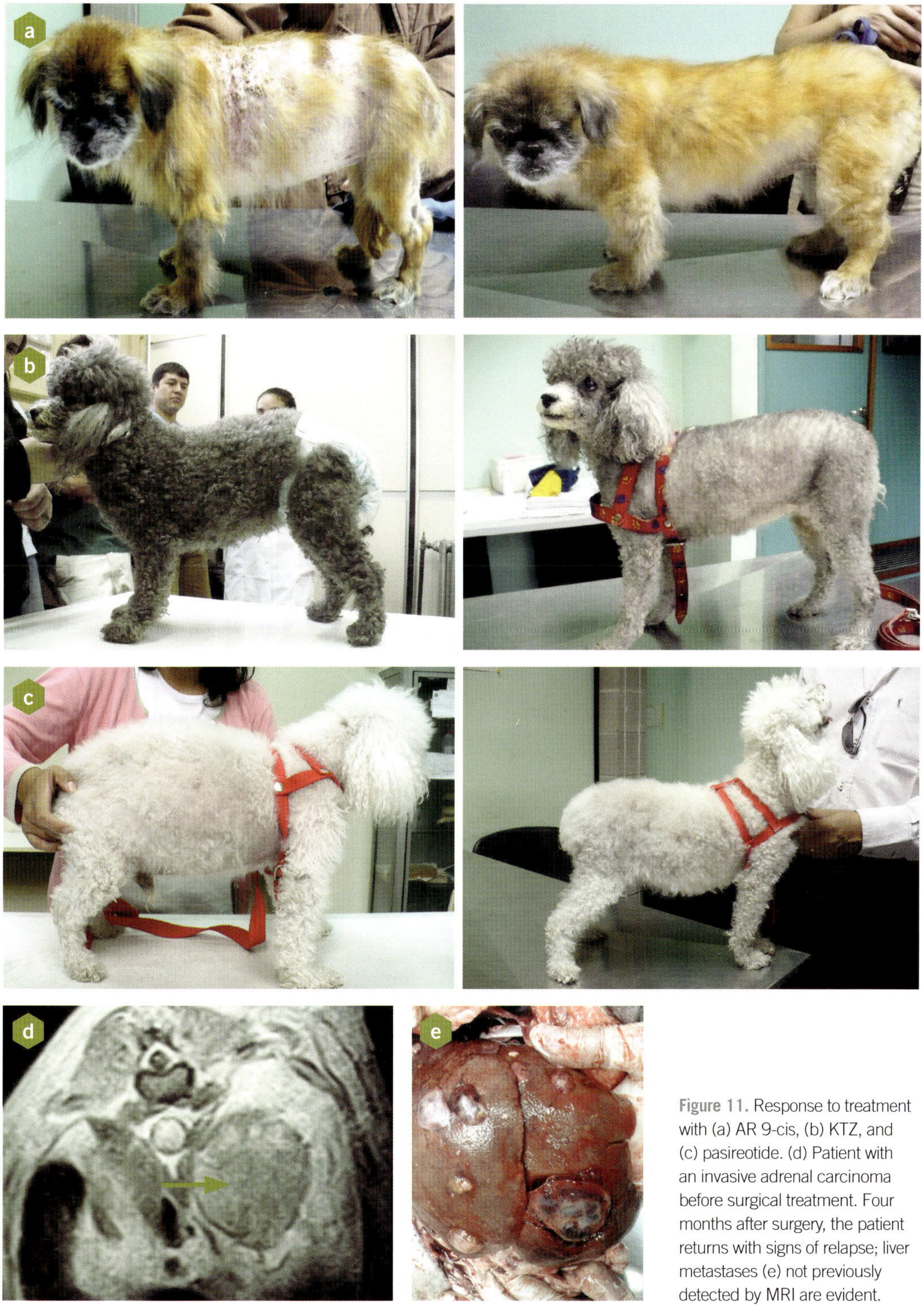

Figure 11. Response to treatment with (a) AR 9-cis, (b) KTZ, and (c) pasireotide. (d) Patient with an invasive adrenal carcinoma before surgical treatment. Four months after surgery, the patient returns with signs of relapse; liver metastases (e) not previously detected by MRI are evident.

ADRENAL INSUFFICIENCY

PHYSIOLOGICAL OVERVIEW

The synthesis of aldosterone (Ads) is more dependent on the concentrations of angiotensin II and circulating K^+ than on the effect of ACTH. The synthesis of Ads requires an increase in the levels of K^+ (which initiates the biosynthetic cascade of this mineralocorticoid) and a decrease in circulating Na^+ levels caused by urinary loss or decrease of blood volume or pressure. The kidney (macula densa) detects these events and releases renin, which converts angiotensinogen into angiotensin II (renin-angiotensin system). This in turn binds to its cell membrane receptor in the glomerular zone, initiating Ads synthesis (Fig. 1). This mineralocorticoid promotes urinary excretion of K^+ and retention of Na^+, chlorine, and water, regulating fluid and electrolyte balance, blood pressure, and blood volume. Increases in circulating Na^+ and Ads levels inhibit the renin-angiotensin system by blocking mineralocorticoid synthesis. In addition, the release of ADH (which dilutes retained Na^+ by retaining solute-free water) inhibits renin synthesis, while the release of atrial natriuretic peptide inhibits the synthesis of Ads and increases Na^+ excretion. [1]

AETIOLOGY

Adrenal insufficiency (AI) is defined as hypofunction of any of the three zones (glomerular, fascicular, reticular) of the adrenal cortex, and can be partial or total, depending on the underlying aetiology. It is usually accompanied by cortisol deficiency, and in some cases decreases in the levels of Ads or androstenedione. [1]

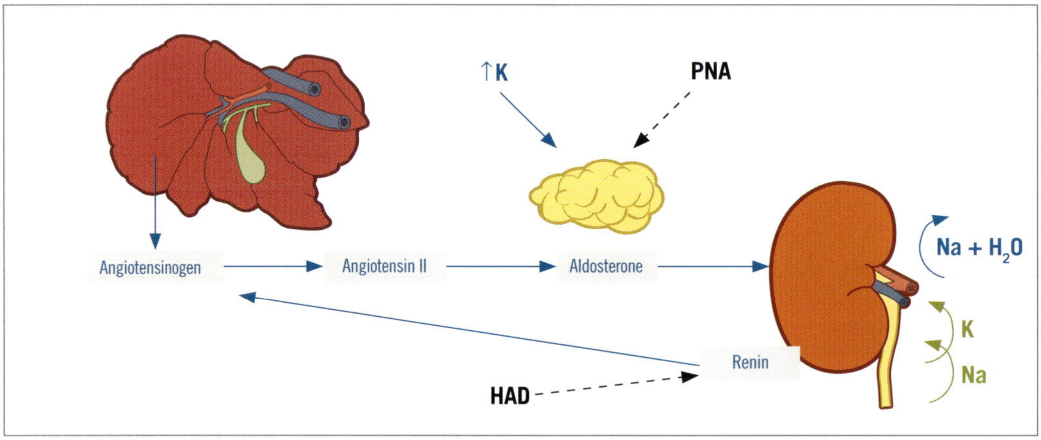

Figure 1. Regulation of Ads. Excretion (green), activation and retention (blue), and inhibition (dashed arrow).

Depending on its origin, [2,3] it is classified as outlined in Table 1:

Table 1. Classification and causes of AI.

Primary	Pituitary insufficiency
▸ Autoimmunity	▸ Lymphocytic hypophysitis
▸ Adrenal hypoplasia	▸ Tumour compression
▸ Infectious	▸ Prolonged corticosteroid therapy
▸ Enzyme deficiency	
▸ Pharmacological	▸ Postadrenalectomy

Primary adrenal insufficiency

Partial or total involvement of the adrenal cortex. Causes:

- Autoimmune: anti-ACTH receptor antibodies and lymphocytic infiltrate. The adrenal cortex is destroyed, while the adrenal medulla is preserved.
- Adrenal hypoplasia: deficiency in transcription factors during the embryonic stage.
- Mycoses, tuberculosis, bacteria: fungi and *Mycobacterium* spp. have a predilection for areas rich in cholesterol, such as the adrenal cortex, promoting the infiltration of lymphocytes, monocytes and macrophages. Bacteria from distant (dental infections, septic arthritis) or contiguous (pyelonephritis) infections cause bacterial adrenalitis (acute).
- Enzymatic deficiency in the synthesis pathway: can affect the adrenal cortex partially or completely, depending on the deficient enzyme (encoded by a mutated gene). A deficiency in the enzyme 3β-hydroxysteroid dehydrogenase (3β-HSD) affects the synthesis of all three hormones (aldosterone, cortisol, and ACTH), whereas a deficiency in 21α-hydroxylase (21α-HXA/CYP21) affects Ads and cortisol. This type of adrenal insufficiency is observed in puppies (congenital) and is characterised by adrenal hyperplasia. This is the result of an increase in the levels of ACTH (inhibition failure), which stimulates the synthesis of the corresponding hormones in the adrenal cortex, a process which is blocked due to enzyme deficiency. This results in an increase in the levels of

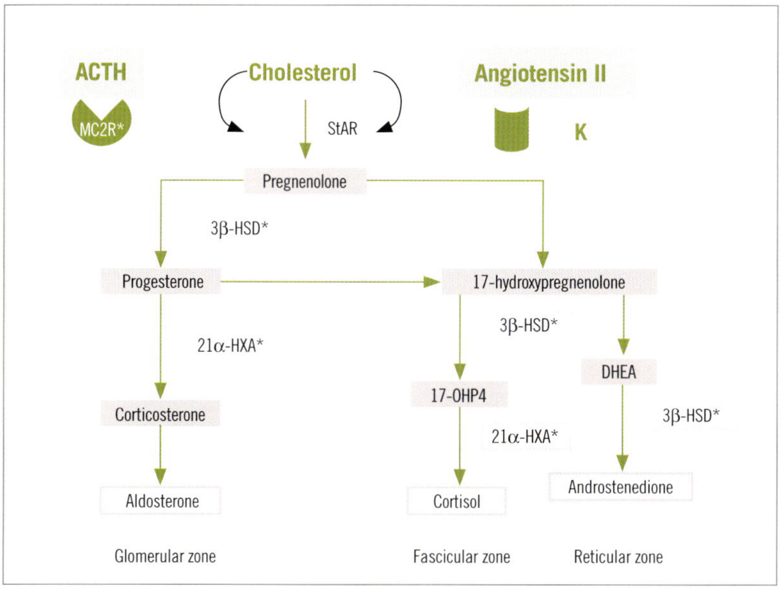

Figure 2. Critical steps in the process of steroid hormone synthesis in the adrenal cortex, the blockade of which (frequent) causes functional deficiency. Critical steps that can be blocked (asterisks). 3β-HSD is present in the 3 regions of the adrenal gland from the beginning of the synthesis process, whereas 21α-HXA is found only in 2 regions, at the end of the process of cortisol and Ads synthesis. A deficit in these enzymes results in increased levels of the precursor.

the metabolic precursors of cortisol and Ads (17-OH progesterone [17-OHP4], progesterone [P4], and pregnenolone) (Fig. 2), and androstenedione. [4,5]

- Pharmacological: caused by anti-steroidogenic drugs (trilostane, ketoconazole, fluconazole, etomidate, aminoglutethimide), which block steroidogenesis or have antineoplastic effect (mitotane).

The first three causes described involve destruction of the AG. This is known as Addison's disease. The other causes are associated with functional failure (hyperplasia of the adrenal cortex may be observed). [2,3]

Pituitary (or secondary adrenal) insufficiency

ACTH secretion is affected. The main causes are lymphocytic hypophysitis, the compressive effect of a nonfunctioning pituitary macroadenoma, and inhibition of the adrenal axis due to prolonged corticosteroid therapy or adrenalectomy due to tumours. Hyposecretion of ACTH affects the synthesis of cortisol and androstenedione, with atrophy of the fascicular and reticular zones. Ads synthesis remains mostly unaffected owing to its regulatory mechanisms. [2,3]

CLINICAL SIGNS

AI is an endocrine disease of low prevalence and is difficult to diagnose. [2,3,6] The most commonly affected species is the dog. It is rare in cats. It usually occurs in young animals, including puppies, but can also be diagnosed in adult animals.

Two forms of presentation are described: acute and chronic. The acute form occurs when the destruction of the adrenal cortex is abrupt (infectious or drug-related), corticosteroid administration is suddenly discontinued, or in case of adrenalectomy, because the adrenal axis is inhibited and the adrenal cortex atrophied, or the pituitary gland is damaged (necrosis due to tumour apoplexy, disconnection from the hypothalamus). The chronic form, which evolves slowly and insidiously, is the most common. Both forms are characterised by non-specific clinical signs (weight loss, cardiovascular and digestive disorders, cachexia) common to other disorders, with which it is often confused. [2,6]

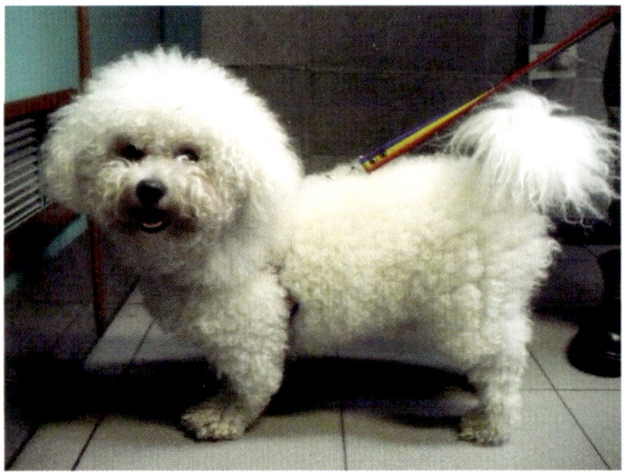

Figure 3. Patient with adrenal insufficiency showing sustained weight loss, lethargy and urine crystallisation.

It is important to obtain a comprehensive medical history in cases in which adrenal insufficiency is suspected, with a particular emphasis on the following:

- Stressful situations (absence of owner, arrival of a new pet, accidents, etc.) temporally related to the appearance of clinical signs (1–7 days before).
- Remission of clinical signs after corticosteroid treatment.
- Formation of crystals in the urine when it dries on the floor (loss of NaCl).
- Any cardiovascular problems (hypotension, bradycardia) the dog may have had, in the absence of an underlying cardiac disease.
- Sporadic convulsive problems not attributable to encephalic or infectious diseases that quickly resolve with corticosteroid treatment.

Table 2. Frequent clinical signs in AI.

Clinical signs	Frequency
Incipient:	
▶ Pruritus	++
▶ Hyperpigmentation	+
▶ Polydipsia/urine crystallisation	+++
▶ Exercise intolerance	++
▶ Bradycardia/hypotension	+++
▶ Gastrointestinal signs	++ (after a stressful situation)
Extreme (Addisonian crisis):	
▶ Cachexia	+++
▶ Abdominal pain, vomiting, diarrhoea	+++
▶ Dehydration and shock	++++
▶ Hypotension and severe bradycardia	++++
▶ Oliguria or anuria	+++
▶ Seizures	+ (assess glycaemia)

Table 3. Clinical signs in puppies with AI due to enzyme deficiency.

Clinical signs	Possible enzyme affected
Severe enzyme deficiency:	
▶ Intrauterine masculinisation of female genitalia.	▶ 21α-HXA deficiency, increased levels of androstenedione and its precursors
▶ Death during birth due to stress	▶ 21α-HXA or 3β-HSD deficiency
Moderate to mild deficiency:	
▶ Pseudohermaphroditism, highly developed clitoris, fusion of vulvar lips resulting in a scrotum-like structure ▶ Male behaviour in females ▶ Genital development inappropriate for age in males (advancement of sexual age) ▶ Anoestrus/absence of first heat	▶ 21α-HXA deficiency, increased levels of androstenedione and its precursors
▶ Growth stunting at 4–5 months of age	▶ 3β-HSD deficiency
▶ Alopecia of perineum and posterior thigh area	▶ 21α-HXA deficiency (due to androstenedione)
▶ Signs of adrenal insufficiency	▶ 21α-HXA or 3β-HSD deficiency

In the chronic phase, clinical signs (Fig. 3) appear as a consequence of the progression of the disease (exhaustion or destruction of the AG). With the decrease in the synthesis of cortisol (firstly) and Ads (subsequently), the metabolic pathways controlled by these hormones (neoglucogenesis, Na^+ and K^+ metabolism) will be altered, affecting various tissues.

Incipient clinical signs (Table 2) include pruritus of nonallergic origin, hyperpigmentation, weight loss with normal appetite, polydipsia, exercise intolerance due to hypotension, and bradycardia. Faced with a stressful event, the AG lacks the capacity to respond to the demand for cortisol and/or Ads, resulting in the appearance of gastrointestinal signs (the most evident clinical signs). In extreme cases (Table 2), patients present with cachexia, abdominal pain, dehydration, and shock with severe hypotension and bradycardia, oliguria or anuria, and seizures due to hypoglycaemia or neuronal dehydration, [2,6] which constitute an Addisonian crisis (medical emergency).

In puppies (Fig. 3), in which the cause may be an enzyme deficiency, [4] the corresponding clinical signs reflect the severity of the deficiency, ranging from ambiguous genitalia (pseudohermaphroditism) due to the action of intrauterine androstenedione to stunted growth at 4–5 months of age (lack of effect of androstenedione on prepubertal bone growth) (Table 3). The owner reports that the puppy grew normally, with proper proportions, up to the aforementioned age. In this case, the differential diagnosis should include growth hormone deficiency and hypothyroidism. Other signs include absent heat and masculinisation in the female (increased territoriality, raising of hindlimb when urinating), early development of the external genitalia in the male or enlargement the clitoris and reduced development of the vulva in the female. [4,5] Over time, the characteristic signs of adrenal insufficiency are observed.

DIAGNOSIS

Laboratory tests

Laboratory data should be interpreted in the context of the clinical signs and medical history in order to facilitate the diagnosis of adrenal insufficiency. Otherwise, these data can lead to confusion, since the findings are not specific to this disorder. The alterations observed are related to a state of adrenal insufficiency.

The following are the most characteristic data to take into account (Table 4): increased haematocrit levels, decreased blood glucose

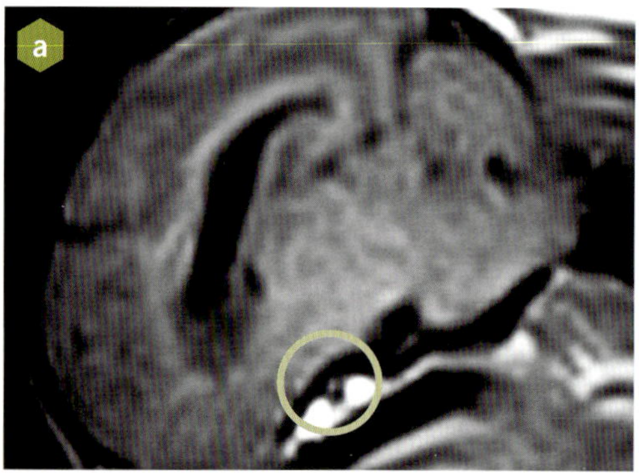

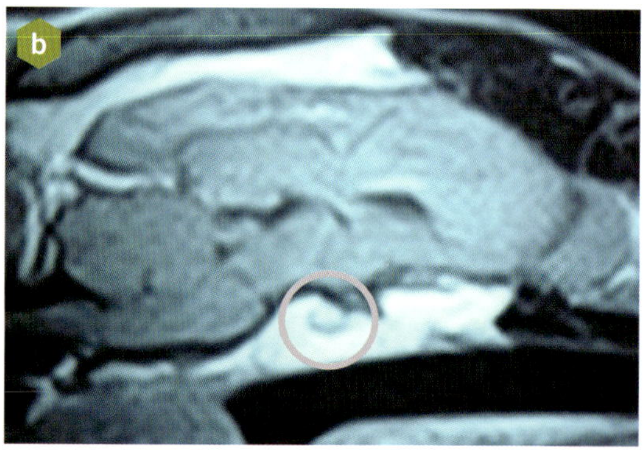

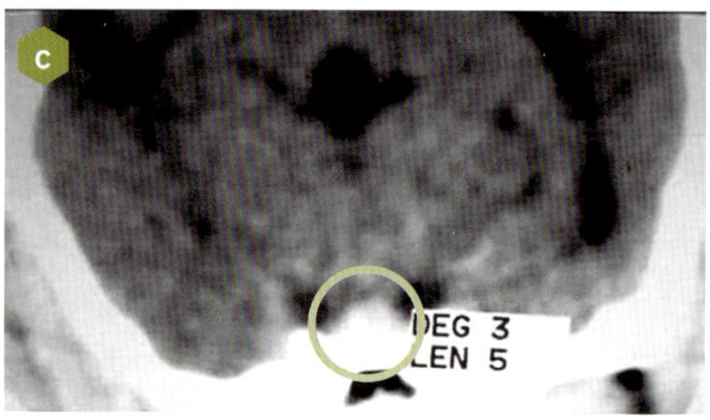

Figure 4. (a and b) MRI and (c) CT in dogs with secondary AI (pituitary insufficiency). (a) Note the small pituitary gland (occupying only part of the sella turcica). (b) The hyperintense pituitary indicates inflammation (characteristic of lymphocytic hypophysitis). (c) A pituitary tumour is visible.

Table 4. Relevant laboratory data and ECGs that are suggestive/diagnostic of AI.

Laboratory data	Status of the variable
Routine laboratory tests (guide):	
▶ Haematocrit	▶ Normal - High (with dehydration and shock)
▶ Glycaemia	▶ At lower limit of normal - Hypoglycaemia (advanced AI)
▶ Urea	▶ Normal - High (depending on stage of AI)
▶ Creatinine	▶ Normal
▶ Ionogram:	
▶ Na^+	▶ Hyponatraemia (AI) - Normonatraemia (pituitary insufficiency or mild AI)
▶ K^+	▶ Hyperkalaemia (AI) - Normokalaemia (liver failure or mild AI)
▶ Na/K ratio	▶ <27/1 (AI) - 27/1–29/1 (suspected AI)
▶ Urine:	
▶ Na^+	▶ Increased urine sodium levels (AI)
▶ K^+	▶ Decreased urine potassium levels (AI)
▶ Specific gravity and sediment	▶ >1020 (loss of NaCl), crystals
Endocrine laboratory tests (confirmatory):	
▶ Stimulation with ACTH:	
▶ Basal cortisol	▶ Normal or hypocortisolaemia
▶ Cortisol 1 hour post-ACTH	▶ Little or no response (<7 µg/dl)
▶ Basal 17-OHP4	▶ High (>0.4 ng/ml), normal, or low *
▶ 17-OHP4 1 hour post-ACTH	▶ Exaggerated response (>2 ng/ml) or low *
▶ Plasma ACTH	▶ High (AI), normal-to-low (pituitary insufficiency)
ECG	▶ Prolongation of P-R interval ▶ Increased amplitude of QRS complex ▶ Increased T-wave amplitude (peak)

* Depending on aetiology: in case of 21α-HXA deficiency, levels will be elevated or normal, and an exaggerated response will be observed after 1 hour. In case of 3β-HSD deficiency or destruction of the cortex, levels will be low and no post-ACTH response will be observed.

levels or hypoglycaemia (more severe cases), and azotaemia with normal creatinine concentration. Ionograms are important (albeit not determinant) to guide the diagnosis towards primary AI. Hyponatraemia, hypochloraemia and hyperkalaemia are characteristic signs, as are alterations in the Na/K ratio. A value <27/1 is indicative of Ads deficiency, whereas values of 27/1 to 29/1 with signs compatible with AI are highly suggestive of this disease. The urine of affected animals contains high Na levels and low K levels. [7] In cases of pituitary insufficiency, the ionogram is usually unaffected, as the glomerular zone continues to be stimulated by angiotensin. [1,2,6,7]

Electrocardiogram (ECG)

The ECG is an important means of evaluating K^+ levels; although circulating concentrations may be normal, increases in the intracellular compartment give rise to ventricular fibrillation and bradycardia. [8] The ECG reveals characteristic alterations (Table 4).

Diagnosis by imaging studies

Of moderate benefit. Ultrasound reveals AG atrophy (advanced AI). In less severe situations, AG size may be normal.

MRI and CT are useful in cases of suspected pituitary insufficiency (Fig. 4).

Endocrine (ACTH stimulation and plasma ACTH measurement)

Definitive diagnosis can only be established following stimulation with ACTH (Fig. 5), which is used to evaluate the responsiveness of the AG. [2,6] Poststimulation measurement of cortisol levels is essential. In addition, 17-OHP-4 is measured in puppies and dogs of up to 2 years of age. A cortisol value <7 μg/dl 1 hour poststimulation is indicative of AI, regardless of the prestimulation concentration. The patient's levels of 17-OHP-4 may be initially elevated (>0.4 ng/ml), showing an exaggerated response 1 hour poststimulation (>2 ng/ml) in cases involving 21α-HXA deficiency. [4,5] If 17-OHP-4 levels do not increase, all three areas of the adrenal cortex will be affected.

Measurement of plasma ACTH allows differentiation between primary AI (high concentration) and pituitary insufficiency (normal or decreased concentration).

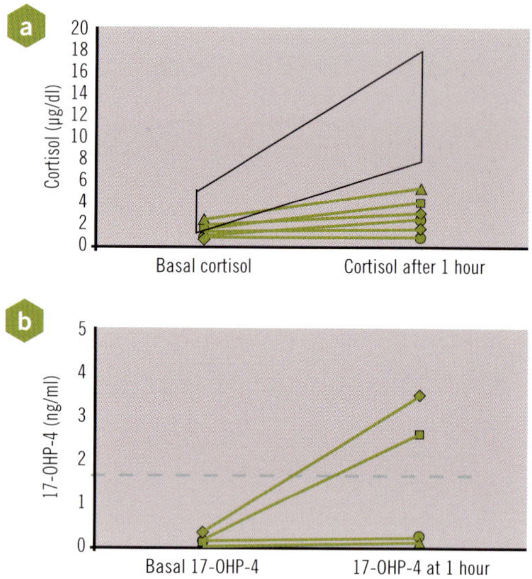

Figure 5. ACTH stimulation test to evaluate (a) cortisol levels pre- and post-ACTH and (b) 17-OHP-4 levels pre- and post-ACTH (4 puppies with AI). (a) The box indicates the expected normal response to cortisol, which may begin at a value within the reference range, but does not exceed 7 μg/dl 1 hour post-ACTH. (b) The dashed line indicates the normal cut-off value post-ACTH for 17-OHP-4.

TREATMENT

Corticosteroid therapy in the management of chronic AI

Hydrocortisone is the treatment of choice owing to its mineralocorticoid effect (1–2 mg/kg/12 hours). Treatment should be monitored by ionogram and ECG, and the dose corrected accordingly. If ionogram or ECG alterations persist, fludrocortisone (0.05–1 mg/day) should be administered in the morning together with hydrocortisone until normalisation of natraemia and the ECG. If hydrocortisone is unavailable, prednisone (same dose as hydrocortisone) can be administered together with fludrocortisone. [2,3,6]

In addition to corticosteroid therapy, it is advisable to add salt to the food or to administer 1 or 2 grains of coarse salt sublingually.

Addisonian crisis

In case an Addisonian crisis is suspected, IV saline solution (0.9 % NaCl) should be administered to correct dehydration and hypotension and to improve natraemia. ECG and emergency laboratory tests (urea, ionogram, blood count, blood glucose) should be performed. Dexamethasone or hydrocortisone (2 mg/kg IV) should be administered if AI is suspected. Once the patient is stabilised, dexamethasone or hydrocortisone treatment should be continued at a dose of 0.5–1 mg/kg/IV or IM every 8 hours until normalisation of the ionogram and ECG. Maintenance treatment should be continued once the patient has recovered from the Addisonian crisis and is stabilised. [2,3,6]

HYPOTHYROIDISM

THYROID AXIS REGULATION

Several characteristics of the HPA axis, thyroid gland and the action of thyroid hormones (TH) must be considered in order to understand their role in different pathologies, and in the diagnosis and treatment of these conditions.

The hypothalamus releases thyrotropin-releasing hormone (TRH), which stimulates the synthesis and release of thyrotropin (TSH) in the anterior pituitary or adenohypophysis. This process is regulated by circulating concentrations of free thyroxine (FT4) (increased levels of which inhibit TSH synthesis). The binding of this hormone to its membrane receptor in the thyroid cell is the first critical step in the synthesis of TH. This is followed by a cascade of events (critical steps): iodine uptake, thyroglobulin (Tg) and thyroperoxidase (TPO) synthesis, incorporation of 4 iodine atoms into the tyrosine residues of Tg to form thyroxine (T4), followed by the formation of triiodothyronine (T3), vacuolisation of thyroid hormones, pinocytosis, and exocytosis (release of T4 and T3 into the peripheral circulation) (Fig. 1). [1,3]

Once released into the bloodstream (T4/T3 ratio of 3:1), 99.9 % of THs are bound to transport proteins. The remaining 0.1 % corresponds to free thyroxine (FT4), which can enter cells in different tissues. Once inside cells, FT4 is deionised to T3 according to the needs of each tissue type. T3 enters the nucleus and binds to its receptor, inducing an adequate response. It also enters mitochondria to regulate thermogenesis. [3,4]

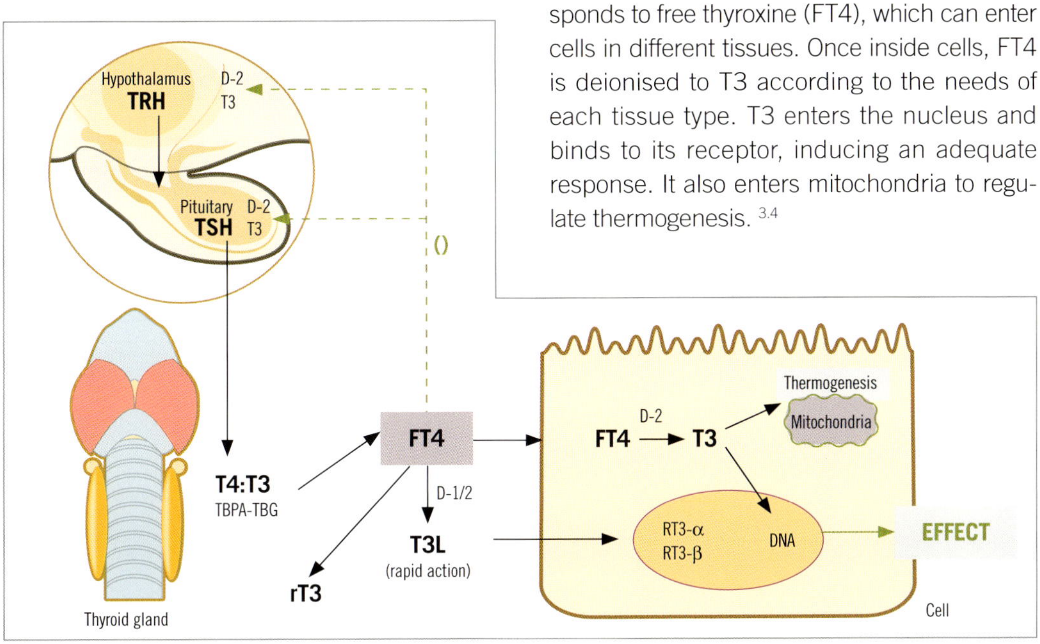

Figure 1. Regulation of thyroid axis, TH, and critical steps.

THs are involved in multiple processes in the body (Table 1) from the moment of fertilisation (they travel through the placenta and play a fundamental role in embryo/foetal development). [5,6]

AETIOLOGY AND CLASSIFICATION

Hypothyroidism (HO) is caused by the insufficient action of TH in its target organs due to reduced TH secretion (destruction of the gland or blockade of the synthesis); a defect in the action of T3 at the level of its nuclear receptor (hormone resistance, usually drug-induced); deficient TSH secretion; or blockade of its action at the level of the thyroid cell (antiTSH receptor antibodies, drugs). [2,4] The aetiology (Table 2) varies between adult animals and puppies; autoimmune thyroiditis is the main cause in adults, whereas the primary cause in puppies is enzyme deficits or defective thyroid development. [6,7,8]

HO is classified according to its clinical manifestation (subclinical and clinical) as well as circulating concentrations of TSH and TH (four stages) (Table 3). [8,9,10] This classification influences treatment. Subclinical HO suggests probable TH deficiency. The process that gives rise to HO is chronic and slow, and involves an initial increase in the levels of antithyroglobulin antibody (ATG) (gland damage), followed by an increase in TSH, triggered in an attempt to maintain an adequate concentration of circulating FT4, and, finally, a decrease in the levels of this hormone due to destruction of the glandular parenchyma (Fig. 2).

Table 1. Main actions of TH.

System, tissue, or organ	Effect
General metabolism (effect on the hepatocyte)	Regulates gluconeogenesis, lipogenesis, and protein synthesis.
Mitochondria	Facultative (body temperature stable at 25 °C) and adaptive (maintains body temperature stable in hot or cold conditions) thermogenesis; oxygen consumption.
Bone and calcium metabolism	Skeletal development and maturation; osteogenesis; calcium regulation; activation of vitamin D (regulates enzyme 1α-hydroxylase); mediator of IGF-1 action and GH release.
Striated and smooth muscle	Sensitivity to nerve stimulation, muscle fibre contraction; regulates endoplasmic reticulum and myoglobin.
Circulatory system	Positive inotropic effect on heart, regulates myoglobin and heart muscle contractility; regulates endothelium and arterial muscle.
Digestive system	Intestinal motility; gallbladder motility (contraction); hydrochloric acid secretion.
Nervous system	Postnatal maturation of the embryonic-foetal nervous system; growth of dendrites and axons (neuronal interconnection); development and maintenance of glial cells; development of Purkinje cells; neuronal metabolism; learning, memory, and behaviour; sensory system; synthesis and maintenance of myelin sheaths; repair of axonal damage.
Hematopoietic system	Regulates erythropoiesis and haemoglobin synthesis; neutrophil chemotaxis.
Immune system	Thymus maturation; thymus selection, T cell maturation and metabolism; chemotaxis.
Reproductive system	▸ Females: stimulates preovulatory LH peak and follicular wave; regulates prolactin. ▸ Gestation: maintains the corpus luteum; T4 and T3 cross the placenta and mediate the development of the embryo and foetus; development of foetal-placental circulation; uterine activity at birth. ▸ Males: spermatogenesis and libido.

IGF1: insulin-like growth factor 1; GH: growth hormone.

Table 2. Main aetiologies of HO.

Stage of life	Causes
Adults	Thyroid: ▶ Autoimmune thyroiditis: lymphocytic infiltration, TSH receptor blockade by antibodies. ▶ Iodine deficiency. ▶ Excess iodine (inhibits thyroid function and predisposes to autoimmune processes). ▶ Non-autoimmune (infectious) thyroiditis: toxoplasmosis, neosporosis, viral or bacterial. Extrathyroid: ▶ Pharmacological: phenobarbital, drugs with antithyroid effects (imidazoles, propranolol), phenobarbital, glucocorticoids. ▶ Pituitary insufficiency (nonfunctioning pituitary adenoma, autoimmune hypophysitis). ▶ Liver failure (decreases synthesis of deiodinases and transport proteins). ▶ Pathologies of the digestive system and malnutrition.
Puppies	Thyroid: ▶ Congenital: lack of thyroid migration (sublingual thyroid), thyroid hypoplasia, defects in the TSH receptor, iodine transporter (NIS), or TPO enzyme. ▶ Postnatal: autoimmune or non-autoimmune thyroiditis. Extrathyroid: ▶ Inadequate HT intake by mother, iodine deficiency, excess iodine (thyroid blockade in foetus or in puppy up to 3 months of age). ▶ Diseases on the digestive tract (megaoesophagus, portosystemic shunt).

Table 3. Classification of HO according to clinical stage and concentrations of TSH and TH.

Clinical stage	Biochemical stage
Subclinical HO	Stage I: ▶ Positive ATG (if autoimmune). ▶ TSH and T4 (total or free): reference values (close to the cut-off limit of normality). ▶ Stimulation with TRH: exaggerated response. ▶ LDL cholesterol may be high. Stage II: ▶ ATG positive (if autoimmune). ▶ Elevated TSH. ▶ T4 (total or free) normal or near lower limit. ▶ LDL cholesterol frequently elevated.
Clinical Ho	Stages III and IV (end of process): ▶ Positive or negative ATG (final stage). ▶ Elevated TSH. ▶ Decreased T4 ▶ Decreased T3 (final stage). ▶ Total cholesterol frequently elevated, elevated LDL. ▶ Triglycerides frequently elevated.

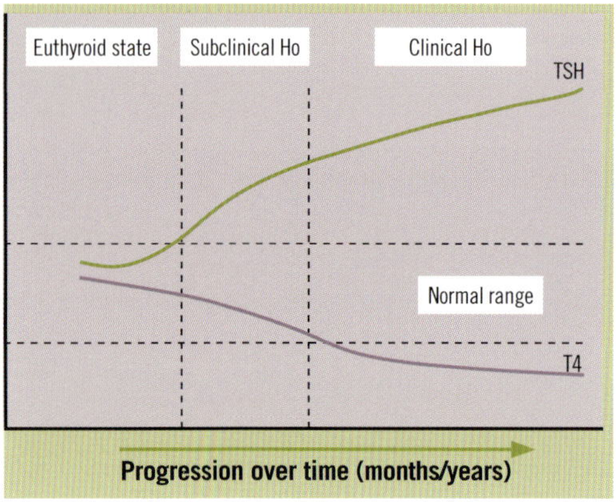

Figure 2. Progression over time from euthyroid state to clinical HO. [9]

Dogs are the most commonly affected species. It is rare in adult cats, and more frequently affects kittens.

CLINICAL SIGNS

Clinical signs vary according to the various actions of TH in the body and depending on the clinical stage and age of the patient. [11,12] Repeated infections (pyoderma and otitis), subfertility (few embryos, embryonic or foetal death, oligospermia), and dyslipidaemia due to increased LDL cholesterol are indicative of subclinical HO.

Clinical signs in clinical HO will depend on the course of the disease and the degree of TH deficiency (Figs. 3–6). The following points should be considered:

- Not all hypothyroid patients are obese. When patients are obese, fat distribution is predominantly subcutaneous (trunk and hips).
- Patients may exhibit hair loss and "rat tail". Hair becomes rough and dull. In long-haired animals, hair length is reduced.
- Alterations in facial expression may be observed: "sad" appearance due to eyelid myxoedema.

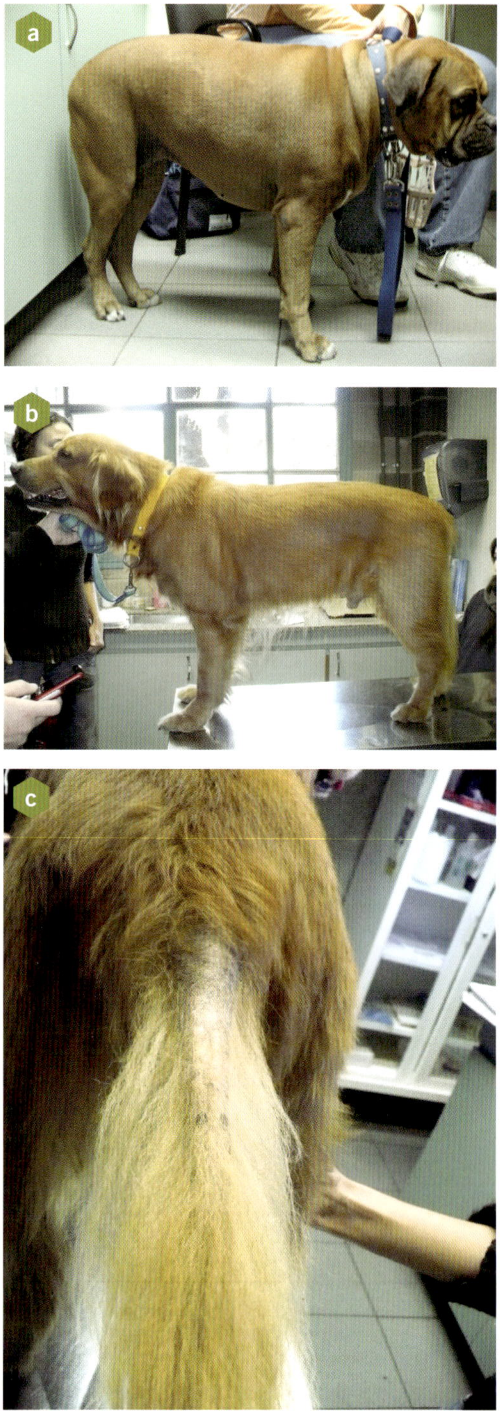

Figure 3. (a) Subclinical and (b and c) clinical hypothyroid patients. (b and c) Very dry, short hair and rat's tail.

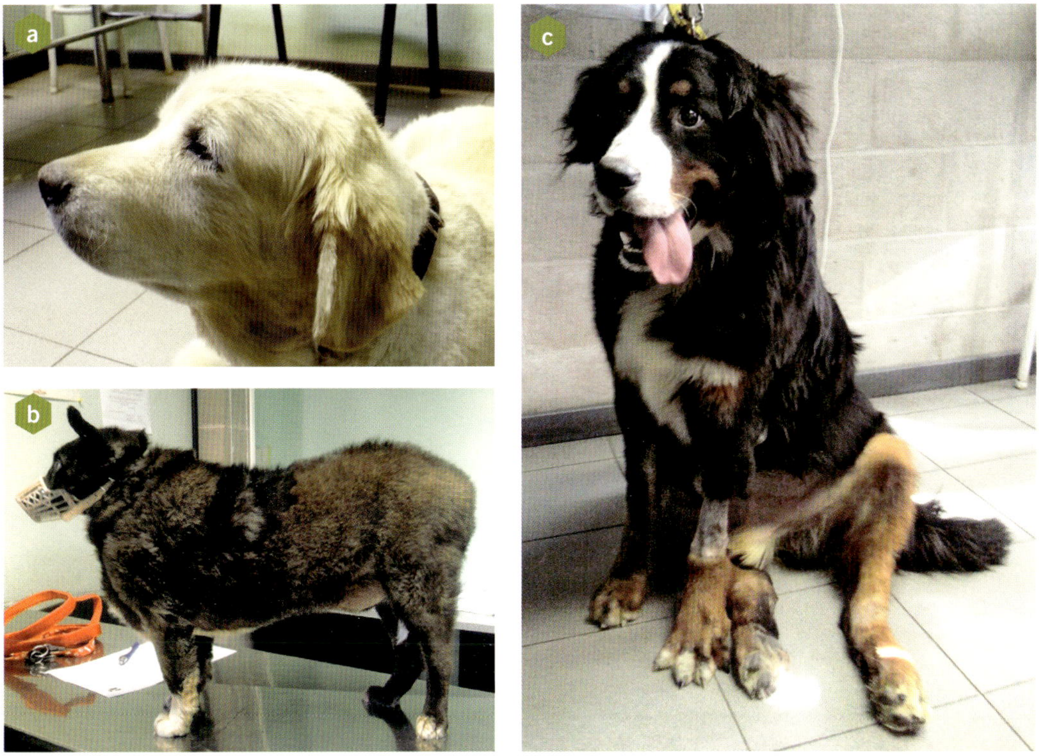

Figure 4. Clinical hypothyroid patients. (a) "Sad" facial expression due to eyelid myxoedema. (b) Loss of coat colour and obesity. (c) Ambulation and mastication difficulties due to myopathy caused by HO.

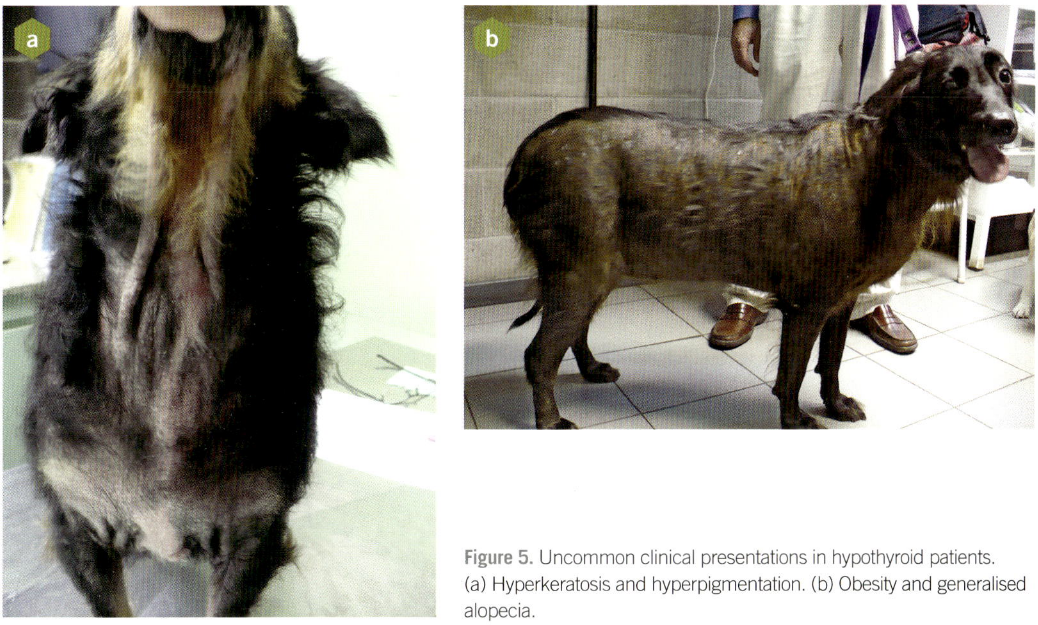

Figure 5. Uncommon clinical presentations in hypothyroid patients. (a) Hyperkeratosis and hyperpigmentation. (b) Obesity and generalised alopecia.

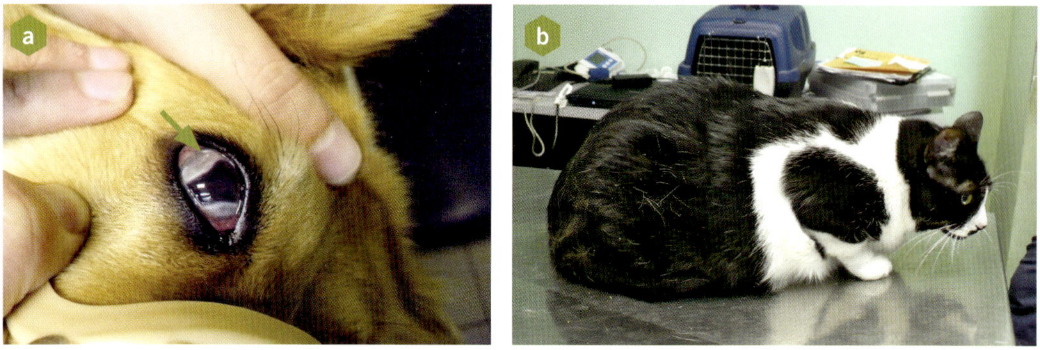

Figure 6. (a) Corneal lipidosis (arrow). (b) Hypothyroid cat: obese, with dry seborrhoea and decreased appetite.

- Temperament may be normal, or patients may be apathetic or exhibit behavioural alterations (e.g. unprecedented aggressiveness).
- An absence of libido (male) or anoestrus may not be observed in all cases. Females may have an anovulatory or oligo-ovulatory oestrous cycle. Fertilisation may occur, although live births will be fewer than expected due to intrauterine death (embryonic/foetal resorption).
- Affected males may present with galactorrhea.
- Cats do not lose hair, but present with seborrhoea and obesity, inappetence, and apathy.

In summary, HO patients are not necessarily obese and lethargic, with bilateral alopecia and seborrhoea. Generally, all these criteria are not fulfilled. It is therefore necessary to consider the entire set of clinical signs, including less obvious

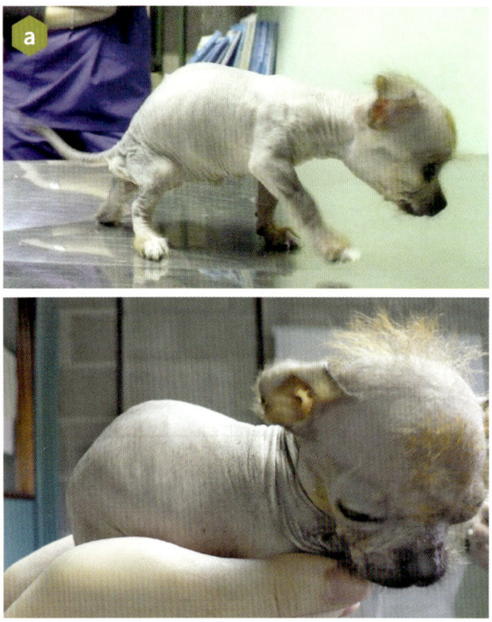

Figure 7. Congenital Ho. (a) A 3-month-old mixed-breed puppy that is smaller than its littermates, has a spherical skull (due to failed parieto-occipital fusion), joint instability, and exhibits disconnection from the environment. (b) A cat that is small for its age, with a defective skull conformation, exhibiting disconnection from the environment.

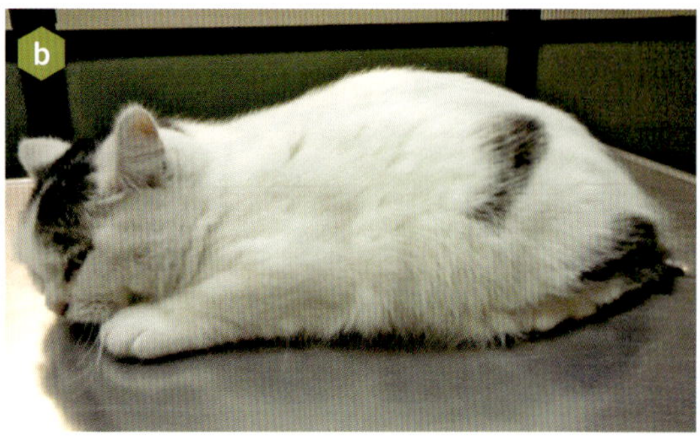

signs or those suggestive of another pathology, such as seizures (e.g. in cases of hypertriglyceridaemia and severe hypercholesterolaemia), corneal lipidosis, recurrent otitis, facial nerve paralysis, malabsorption syndrome, biliary sludge, etc. Correct interpretation of the clinical signs will enable a presumptive diagnosis of HO, after which the appropriate additional studies required for diagnostic confirmation should be performed.

Clinical manifestations in puppies are more marked (Fig. 7). Affected puppies are underweight and smaller at birth (effects already observable in utero by ultrasound). They have spherical, abnormally proportioned skulls, with no parieto-occipital fusion and a shortened nose. They lack a sucking reflex and are rejected by the mother, have a cleft palate, and display reduced activity and disconnection from the environment (no playing behaviour). In addition, they have a reduced growth rate and are therefore smaller than their littermates, show hearing problems, delays in walking, and delayed hair growth and tooth eruption. Other notable features include absence of the patella, bone immaturity, and osteopenia, which is evident on radiographs. [6,13,14,15,16,17]

DIAGNOSIS

Routine laboratory tests to guide diagnosis

Except for changes in the lipid profile, routine laboratory tests (Table 4) reveal no alterations, or alterations that are not typical or indicative of HO. In advanced cases, normocytic normochromic anaemia and increased AI due to hepatic steatosis may be observed. [18]

Lipid metabolism is altered in the early stages, and is evident from the first stages of the disease. It is advisable to measure LDL (low density lipoprotein) cholesterol, which increases due to reduced expression of the LDL receptor in hepatocytes regulated by T3. Since the predominant fraction in dogs and cats is HDL (high density lipoprotein) cholesterol (in 70 % of cases), with an HDL/LDL ratio of 3:1, [19] alterations in this ratio (<2.5:1) are caused by an increase of LDL cholesterol. Lipid profile evaluation should include total cholesterol, HDL, LDL and triglycerides (Table 4).

Table 4. Laboratory tests necessary for diagnostic guidance and definitive diagnosis of Ho.

Laboratory tests	Expected results
Complete blood count	▶ Normochromic normocytic anaemia (advanced stages).
Routine biochemistry tests	▶ Elevated alkaline phosphatase (AP) (liver steatosis). ▶ Normal or elevated total cholesterol (depending on stage of HO). ▶ LDL cholesterol usually elevated. ▶ HDL/LDL ratio <2.5/1. ▶ Elevated triglycerides in severe cases.
Endocrine biochemical analyses	▶ ATG * (positive in autoimmune thyroiditis). ▶ TSH. * ▶ Specific FT4 * (by chemiluminescence). ▶ Total T4 * (if FT4 test not available). ▶ Stimulation with TRH * (basal TSH + TSH 15–20 minutes).

* See Table 3.

Confirmatory laboratory tests

To confirm diagnosis (Table 4), it is necessary to measure TSH and specific free T4 (chemiluminescence method) together with ATG. It is important to factor in any medication taken by the patient that may affect thyroid function, as well as any age-associated alterations in total T4 and FT4.[2,12,20] If TSH and FT4 are within the reference range, but close to cut-off values, and the patient is positive for ATG, with elevated LDL cholesterol levels and alterations in gland morphology as revealed by ultrasound, a TRH stimulation test should be performed. This involves IV administration of a complete vial of TRH, after which blood is extracted to measure basal TSH levels. TSH levels >0.5 ng/ml in blood samples collected after 20 minutes are suggestive of HO.[10]

For diagnosis of HO, the following parameters should be taken into account:

- TSH is the best and most sensitive indicator of the status of the thyroid axis. Elevated TSH levels are diagnostic for HO (lack of inhibition of the thyroid axis), regardless of FT4 values.
- FT4 levels provide an indication of the individual's thyroid status (euthyroid, hypothyroid, or hyperthyroid), thyroid function, the extent of thyroid gland involvement, and T4 supply to tissues. However, a normal value does not rule out the disease, which may be in the subclinical stage (elevated TSH).
- ATG should be evaluated as an early marker of thyroid damage. If the result is positive, and TSH and FT4 concentrations are normal, a TRH stimulation test should be performed.

Table 5. TTV in adult dogs and cats.

Weight	TTV (ml)
1–10 kg (dog)	0.05–0.1 (<5 kg); 0.15–0.2 (5–10 kg)
<5 kg (cat)	0.05–0.2
10–20 kg (dog)	0.25–0.8
20–30 kg (dog)	0.8–1.7
>40 kg (dog)	1.52.2

Diagnosis by imaging studies

Ultrasound is the method of choice. Total thyroid volume (TTV) should be calculated using the following formula:[21,22]

TTV: length × thickness × width × 0.523 (correction factor). TTV is the result of the sum of the volumes of the right (LLV) and left (RLV) lobes. Ultrasound provides information on the size (Table 5) and appearance of the thyroid gland, as well as the presence of nodules or thyroid tumours (Fig. 8).

In puppies, in addition to ultrasound, it is important to perform radiographs of the paw, stifle, and lumbar spine (to evaluate bone maturation), as well as gamma camera scintigraphy, which can provide information on the underlying aetiology (a lack of radiotracer uptake indicates a iodine transport deficiency; uptake can be indicative of defective organification; sublingual uptake is indicative of ectopic thyroid) (Fig. 9).

TREATMENT

Treatment should be adapted to the individual patient and the physiological situation. Factors to take into account include heart or kidney disorders, whether the animal will mate or is pregnant, and the patient's age (a lower dose is recommended in geriatric dogs).

The goal of treatment (levothyroxine) is to normalise the thyroid axis and levels of circulating FT4. Levothyroxine is usually given every 24 hours (as a solution).[3,4,23] The dose varies according to the disease stage (subclinical or clinical) and should be administered following fasting (food should be provided 1 hour after treatment). The objective is to achieve FT4 values at the upper limit and TSH values at the lower limit, thus avoiding periods of low FT4.

Doses of 2–5 µg/kg/day (subclinical HO) or 10–20 µg/kg/day (clinical HO) are indicated, beginning with the lowest dose, which is then increased while monitoring the patient until an

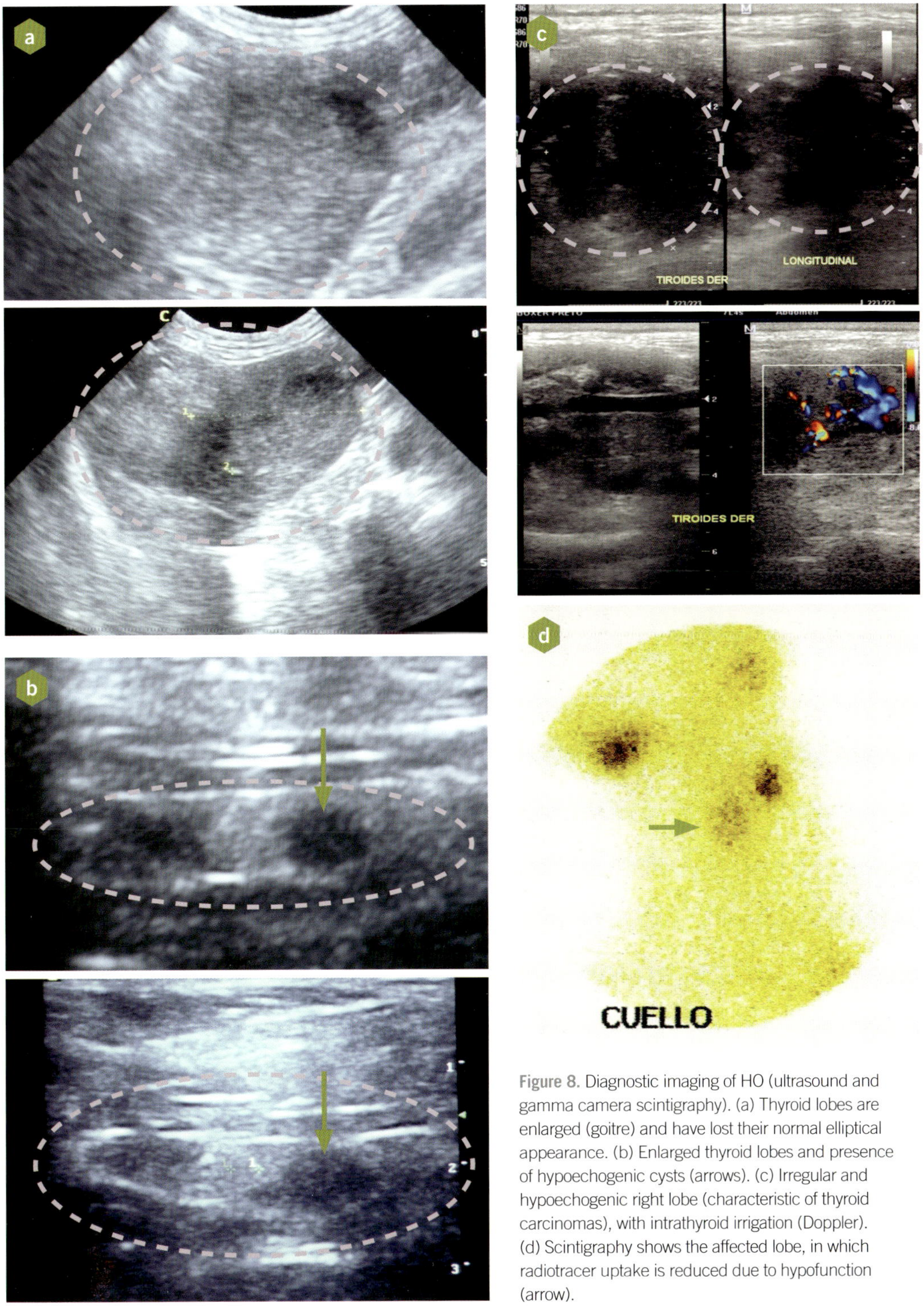

Figure 8. Diagnostic imaging of HO (ultrasound and gamma camera scintigraphy). (a) Thyroid lobes are enlarged (goitre) and have lost their normal elliptical appearance. (b) Enlarged thyroid lobes and presence of hypoechogenic cysts (arrows). (c) Irregular and hypoechogenic right lobe (characteristic of thyroid carcinomas), with intrathyroid irrigation (Doppler). (d) Scintigraphy shows the affected lobe, in which radiotracer uptake is reduced due to hypofunction (arrow).

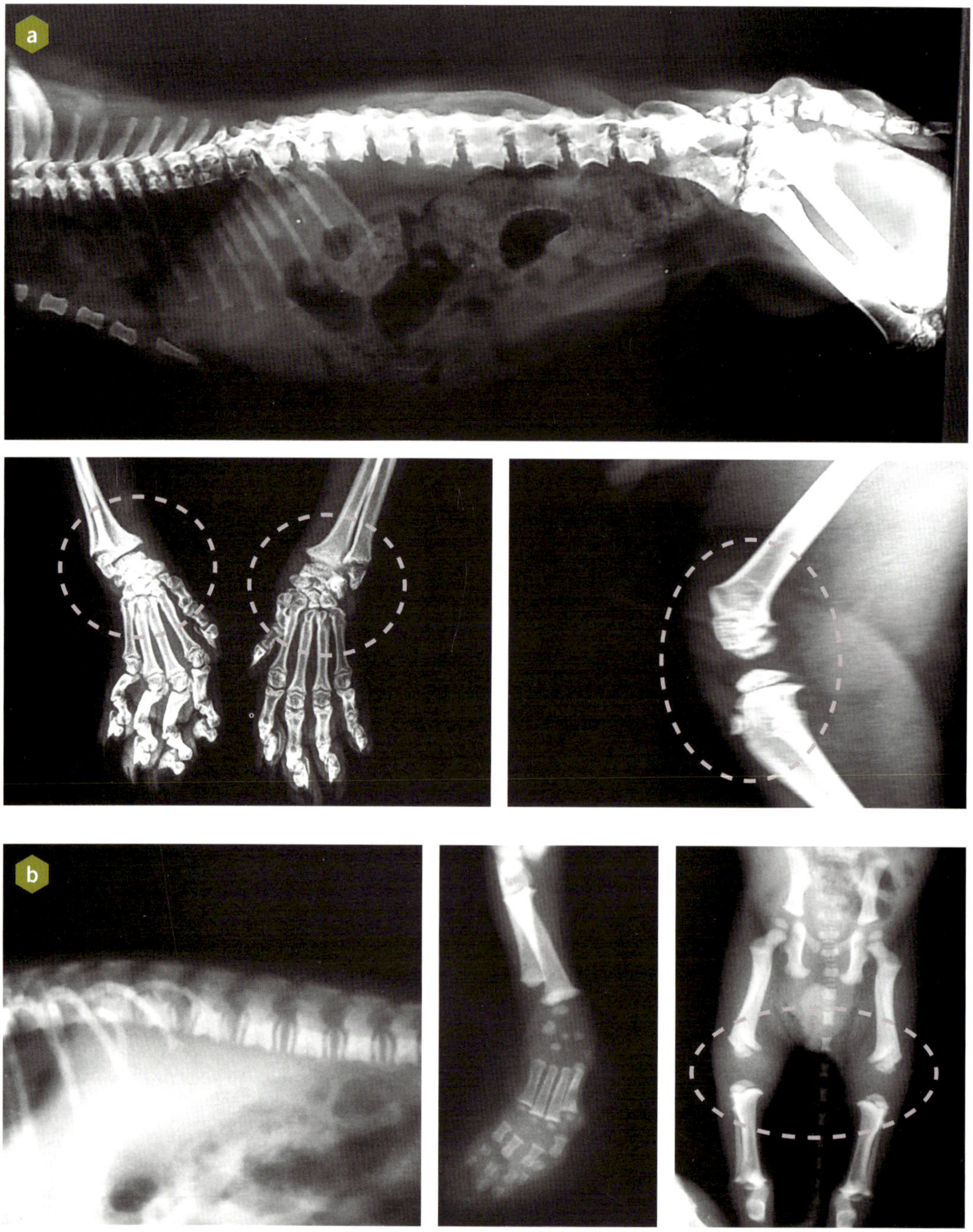

Figure 9. Diagnosis by imaging in cases of congenital HO. (a) Vertebral immaturity (articular facets not fused to the vertebral body), delayed maturation in the radioulnar and carpal areas (no fusion or articulation of the styloid process of the ulna) in a cat of 1.5 years of age. (b) A 3-month-old dog exhibiting skeletal immaturity in the spine and paw (note the carpal bones, the radius with poor development of its distal epiphysis, and the ulna; their image corresponds to that of a 30- to 40-day-old puppy), and in other bones. Note also the absence of the patella.

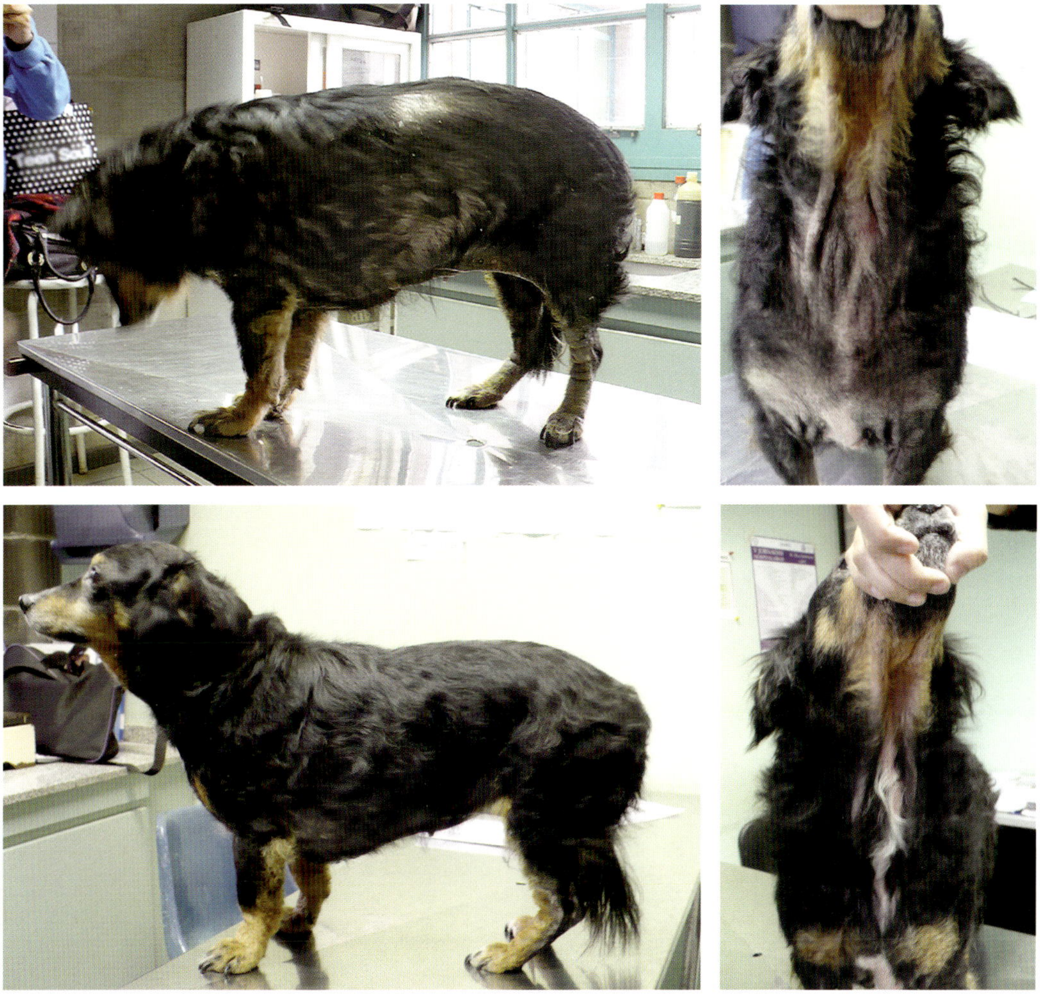

Figure 10. Treatment with levothyroxine in a 3-month-old dog that received 5 µg/kg/day in a single dose (heart disorder). Note hair growth in affected areas and the disappearance of hyperpigmentation and hyperkeratosis.

appropriate dose is reached. In senior animals or those with heart or kidney disorders, it is preferable to begin with the subclinical HO dose and to allow FT4 to approach the lower limit. In puppies it is advisable to begin treatment immediately at a dose of 5–10 µg/kg/day (Fig. 10), even if HO has not been diagnosed, since the sequelae of TH deficiency (neurological or bone) can be irreversible.

Treatment monitoring is carried out every 2 months after starting levothyroxine treatment at the indicated dose; blood samples should be extracted 4 or 6 hours after administration (the moment of maximum absorption).[23,24] Depending on the value obtained the dose is adjusted (increased by 25 %) or not. In patients with heart or kidney disorders, the function of these organs should be evaluated before increasing the dose. If appropriate, the dose should be increased by only 10 % until the next evaluation.

HYPERTHYROIDISM

INTRODUCTION

Hyperthyroidism (H+) is characterised by increased autonomous or independent production of TH, without TSH regulation. Contrary to the situation in HO, H+ is characterised by the inhibition of both the thyroid axis and TSH (very low or undetectable levels). The supply of T4 to tissue is increased, augmenting the effects of the hormone, increasing the activity of certain metabolic pathways (gluconeogenesis, lipolysis, and proteolysis), activating bone resorption, and increasing tissue oxygen consumption, and hence thermogenesis. Owing to the excess of TH, sensitivity to the action of catecholamines and to the autonomic nervous system is increased in cardiac and arterial muscle, smooth gastrointestinal muscle (increased motility), and the kidneys. [1,2,3]

While more prevalent in cats, H+ can occur in dogs, usually as a consequence of a thyroid tumour. [2,4,5,6] It is more frequent in cats aged >8–9 years, and less common at younger ages. [2,4,7] The age of presentation in dogs is variable and depends on the underlying aetiology, which in this author's experience is usually of autoimmune origin in young animals (<4 years of age) and associated with thyroid tumours in adults (>5 years of age). [5]

CLASSIFICATION AND AETIOLOGY

H+ is classified as subclinical (HT close to the upper limit with TSH inhibited) or clinical, [1,8,9,10] and develops progressively (Fig. 1). Clinical signs in subclinical H+ are nonspecific and erratic. Most affected patients have diabetes mellitus, which mimics subclinical H+. In cats, continuous weight loss and the need for high doses of insulin to normalise blood glucose are indicative of H+.

Aetiological classification (Table 1):

- Thyroid adenoma: main cause of H+ in cats. This is caused by mutations in genes encoding the TSH receptor or G protein, [11,12,13,14,15,16,17,18,19] resulting in permanent activation of the HT synthesis pathway and the RAS oncogene, which in turn gives rise to increased mitogenesis and the development of a toxic nodular goitre (the other thyroid lobe is inhibited) or a toxic multinodular goitre affecting one or both lobes (bilateral or diffuse toxic goitre).

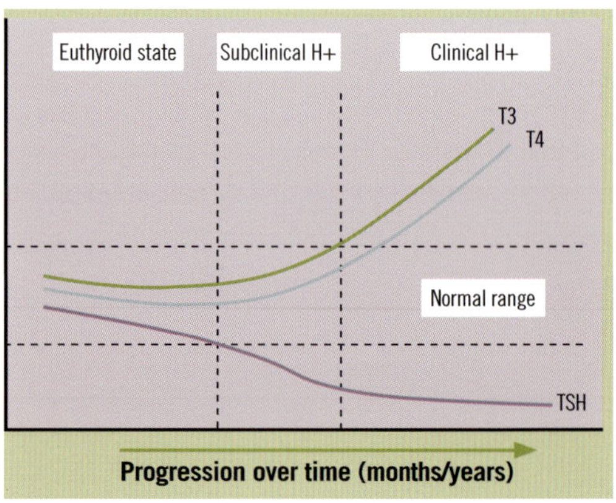

Figure 1. Progression from euthyroid state to clinical HO.[1]

- Autoimmune: in contrast to the situation in humans, the presence of TSH receptor–stimulating antibodies in cats [2,11,12,20] has not been demonstrated, but has also not been ruled out. Few studies have been performed in dogs, although those diagnosed show high levels of ATG and FT4, and decreased levels of TSH. This clinical picture is characterised by diffuse toxic goitre.
- Iodine-induced H+: due to the excess of iodide ions, the gland acts autonomously, synthesising and releasing greater amounts of TH to remove the excess iodine. [21,22,23] Moreover, the excess of iodine predisposes the patient to autoimmune processes and thyroid adenoma.
- Well-differentiated follicular thyroid carcinoma: this is the main cause of H+ in dogs, and occurs less frequently in cats. [5,11,24] In dogs, 10 % of cases of follicular thyroid carcinomas are associated with concomitant H+. [6]
- Ectopic thyroid: the remnants of the embryonic thyroid that persist after migration during the embryonic stage can mutate, giving rise to toxic adenoma or follicular thyroid carcinoma. [2,5,7,25] These neoplastic embryonic remnants are frequently found in the anterior mediastinum (within the thorax) or at the base of the tongue. The thyroid lobes may appear normal, or can be atrophied and inhibited. In some cases, one or both of the thyroid lobes, as well as the embryonic remnants, are simultaneously affected.

DIAGNOSIS

Clinical signs

Clinical signs (Table 2) depend on the course of the disease. In the subclinical stage, cats exhibit [8,9] cyclical loss and gain of weight, alternating periods of normal and increased defecation frequency, and increased hair loss and regrowth.

Table 1. Main aetiologies of H+.

Species	Causes
Cats	▸ G-protein mutation. ▸ Toxic unilateral adenoma. ▸ Toxic multinodular goitre (unilateral or bilateral). ▸ Thyroid follicular carcinoma. ▸ Dietary excess of iodine (iodine-induced). ▸ Autoimmune: TSH receptor-stimulating antibody (under discussion). ▸ Embryological ectopic thyroid.
Dog	▸ Differentiated follicular thyroid carcinoma. ▸ Autoimmune. ▸ Embryological ectopic thyroid.

Table 2. Frequent clinical signs in hyperthyroid cats and dogs.

Species	Clinical signs
Cats	▸ Diabetes mellitus (subclinical). ▸ Cycles of weight loss and gain (subclinical). ▸ Increased frequency of defecation. ▸ Excessive hair replacement (increased loss and regrowth). Bristly, uneven, and dull hair. ▸ PU/PD. ▸ PP (5 % with anorexia). ▸ Progressive weight loss. ▸ Behavioural changes, fearfulness, hyperexcitation (in some cases). ▸ Tachycardia-arterial hypertension. ▸ Fractures due to osteoporosis (uncommon). ▸ Palpation of unilateral or bilateral goitre in the thyroid area of the neck or at the base of the neck.
Dog	▸ Weight loss. ▸ Chronic hyperthermia. ▸ Dry hair, loss of hair. ▸ Tachycardia-arterial hypertension. ▸ Tachypnoea. ▸ Palpation of tumour mass in the thyroid area of the neck. ▸ Palpation of bilateral goitre (autoimmune).

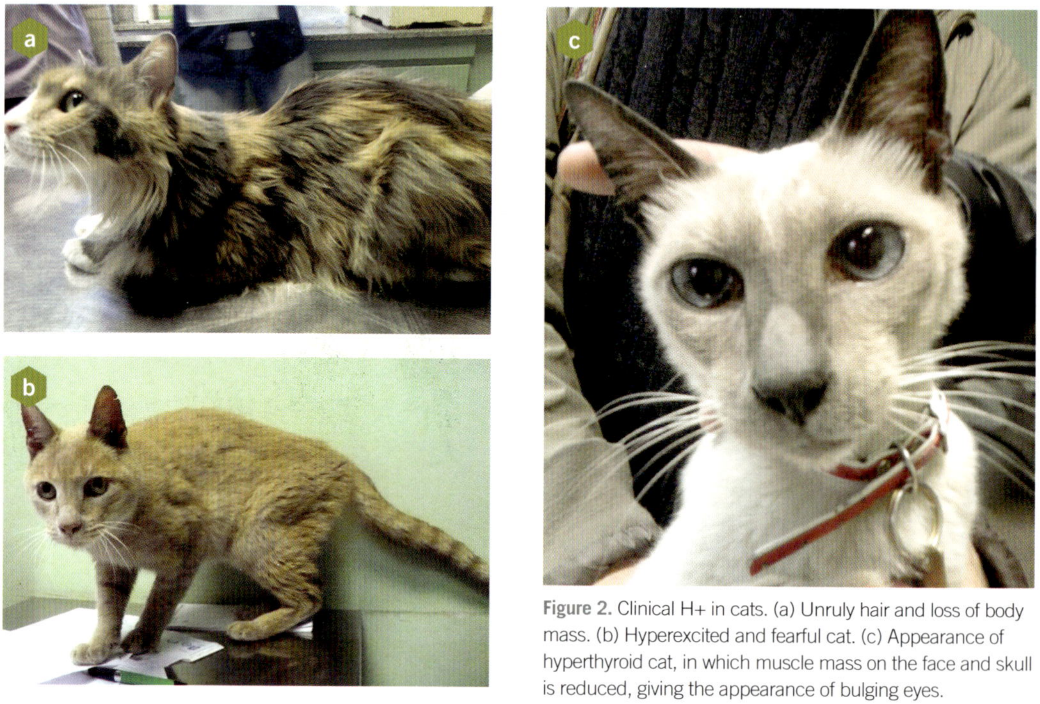

Figure 2. Clinical H+ in cats. (a) Unruly hair and loss of body mass. (b) Hyperexcited and fearful cat. (c) Appearance of hyperthyroid cat, in which muscle mass on the face and skull is reduced, giving the appearance of bulging eyes.

If early diagnosis is not established and T4 levels are persistently moderately elevated or are at the upper cut-off limit, the patient may develop diabetes mellitus (presenting complaint).

In the clinical phase, the most common clinical signs (Fig. 2) are loss of weight and muscle mass, constant hair replacement (alopecia is not observed unless hair is pulled out due to anxiety), behaviour changes, fearfulness (hyperexcitation is uncommon), polyuria, polydipsia, and polyphagia (PU/PD/PP) (about 5 % may present with anorexia), tachycardia, and hypertension. On examination of the thyroid area, one or both of the enlarged lobes can be palpated. The enlarged thyroid descends due to gravity, resting at the base of the neck where it joins the thorax. [2,8]

Dogs (Fig. 3) present with hair loss, dry, thin hair, mild alopecia, hyperthermia, tachycardia, and arterial hypertension. It is possible to palpate the tumoural lobe (3–10 cm) or both enlarged lobes during examination of the thyroid area (autoimmune aetiology).

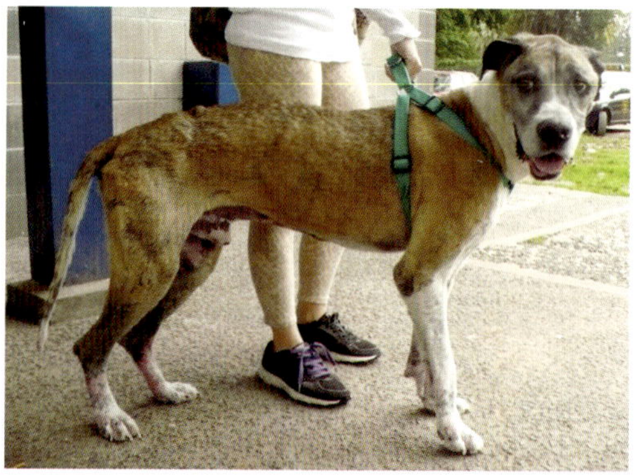

Figure 3. Dog with H+ due to left follicular thyroid carcinoma (palpable mass measuring about 10 cm). Coat colour loss, dry hair, and alopecia in different areas, as well as loss of muscle mass and weight, tachycardia, hypertension and polyphagia.

Table 3. Laboratory findings indicative of H+.

Laboratory analyses	Expected results
Routine biochemistry tests	▸ Elevated ALT/GPT. ▸ Elevated GGT. ▸ Normal total cholesterol at the lower limit. ▸ Normal glucose at the upper limit or fasting hyperglycaemia (very common). ▸ Glucose >220 mg/dl. ▸ Urea and creatinine levels at upper limit of normal or elevated (due to muscle atrophy or concurrent renal failure). ▸ Calcium levels normal or elevated (5–8 % of cases). ▸ Increased AP levels in bone.
Endocrine biochemical tests	▸ TSH inhibited or suppressed (not detectable). ▸ Specific FT4 and total T4 elevated or at the upper limit of normal in subclinical cases. ▸ Elevated T3 (very advanced stages). ▸ ATG positive (in dogs). ▸ Inhibition with T3: does not inhibit T4 (indicated in subclinical cases).

Routine laboratory tests to guide diagnosis

Routine laboratory tests are useful to detect H+ (especially subclinical H+). Levels of ALT/GPT and GGT should be analysed; these are usually elevated since they are involved in gluconeogenesis, proteolysis, and TH catabolism in the liver. [2,3,4,26] It is also important to evaluate levels of glucose, total cholesterol, urea, and creatinine (Table 3).

Confirmatory laboratory tests

Definitive diagnosis is established by measuring levels of T4, FT4, and T3 (which is of diagnostic relevance in H+), which are generally increased or at the upper cut-off limit. TSH levels will be decreased or undetectable in tests. [27,28] If T4 concentrations are close to the upper cut-off, and TSH levels are decreased (suspicion of subclinical H+), a T3 inhibition test should be performed, [29] especially if gamma camera scintigraphy is unavailable.

This test is based on the fact that, if the thyroid axis is not inhibited and the TH concentrations recorded are random or due to another cause, the thyroid axis will be inhibited by administering T3 (20 µg PO), which results in decreased T4 concentrations at 2 and 4 hours. By contrast, in the case of subclinical H+, the axis is already inhibited, and therefore T4 will not decrease after T3 administration. [27,29]

Dogs may present with transient biochemical H+, characterised by increased T4 levels and normal or elevated TSH levels. This can be caused by the following: [30,31]

- Presence of antibodies that interfere with the T4 test, resulting in higher values.
- Rupture of thyroid follicles due to infectious causes (toxoplasmosis, neosporosis).
- Initial stages of autoimmune thyroiditis (destruction of follicles or transient thyroid stimulation).

In these cases, patients should not be treated for H+; hormone levels should be re-evaluated every month. Generally, T4 concentrations fall and the patient develops HO. In cases involving an infectious aetiology, T4 usually returns to its normal values once the cause has been treated and thyroid follicles are repaired.

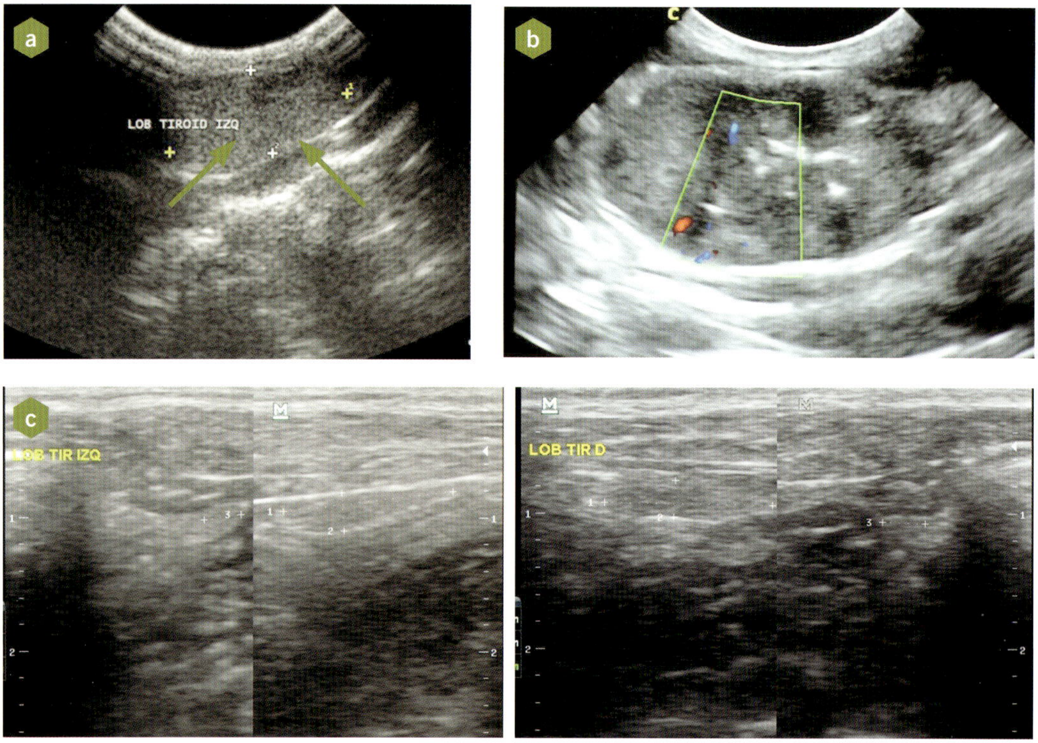

Figure 4. Ultrasound diagnosis in hyperthyroid patients. (a) Image showing nodular presentation, resulting in altered lobe shape (unilateral toxic nodule) (arrows). (b) Appearance of follicular carcinoma, with positive Doppler signal. (c) Increased size of both lobes (toxic bilateral goitre).

Diagnosis by imaging studies

Ultrasonography and gamma camera scintigraphy [2,13,32,33] are complementary tests, the results of which will determine the treatment of choice. Ultrasound reveals the morphology of the thyroid lobes, and whether the goitre affects one or both lobes (adenomas, nodules, or carcinomas) (Fig. 4). Ultrasound cannot be used to detect ectopic thyroid tissue.

Gamma camera scintigraphy can be used to assess thyroid gland function based on radiotracer uptake, which is classified as follows: excess uptake (hyperfunction with high levels of functional activity); normal uptake (normal function); or decreased uptake (the thyroid lobe is inhibited and shows low or null functionality). Scintigraphy can be employed to determine the

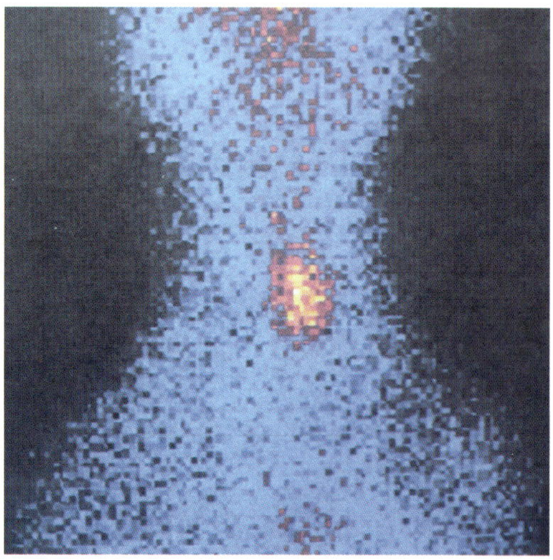

Figure 5. Gamma camera scintigraphy image of a cat with a unilateral toxic nodule (follicular adenoma). The other lobe is completely inhibited (very little uptake).

presence of intrathoracic or sublingual ectopic thyroid, and whether excess uptake occurs in one (toxic unilateral adenoma or follicular carcinoma) or both (diffuse toxic goitre) lobes (Fig. 5). In iodineinduced H+ both lobes show normal or low uptake; because the lobes are saturated with iodine, radiotracer uptake is prevented.

Although ultrasound can indicate that both thyroid lobes are morphologically normal, they may be hyperfunctioning or contain functioning ectopic thyroid remnants, hence the need for gamma camera scintigraphy.

Based on the data obtained from both tests, a definitive treatment can be selected.

TREATMENT

Treatment involves four basic steps:

- Reestablishment of a euthyroid state using antithyroid drugs (methylmercaptoimidazole [MMI] or methimazole, carbimazole, propylthiouracil), followed by definitive treatment once the patient has stabilised. [34,35]
- Control of heart rate, high blood pressure, and kidney function. [3]
- Reduction of iodide ion intake (substitution with a low-iodine diet or a homemade diet if a commercial diet is not commercially available) until final treatment. [22,23,36]

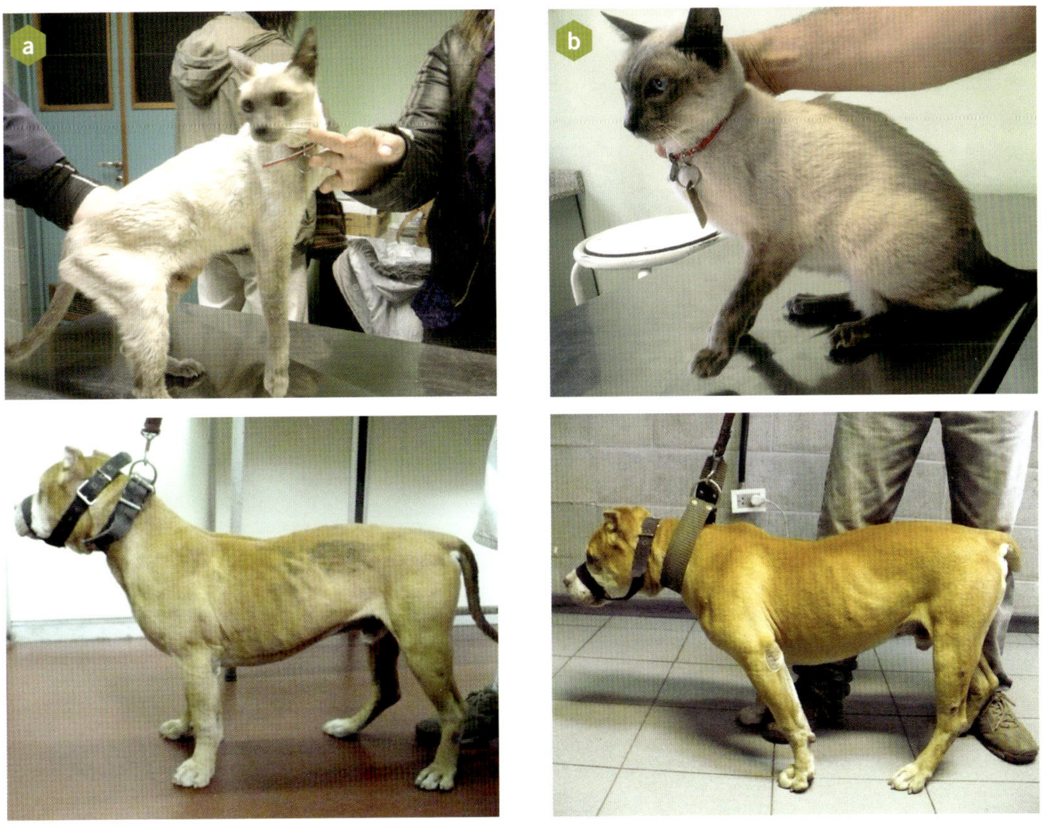

Figure 6. Evolution of two patients in a (a) hyperthyroid and (b) euthyroid state 2 months after receiving MMI treatment, with normalisation of FT4, T4, T3, and TSH concentrations.

- Institute a definitive treatment according to drug availability and owner compliance once the patient is euthyroid:
  - Ablative dose of ^{131}I (in cases of diffuse toxic goitre, ectopic thyroid, after surgery for follicular thyroid carcinoma or if it recurs postoperatively). [2,7,13]
  - Unilateral thyroidectomy in cases of unilateral nodule or thyroid carcinoma. [35,37]
  - Antithyroid drugs if the ablative dose cannot be achieved with ^{131}I, or evaluation of the possibility of a total thyroidectomy (preserving the parathyroid gland). [7,35,37]

MMI or methimazole is the most widespread drug treatment, and is available in most countries. Carbimazole belongs to the same family as MMI, but its availability is more limited. The initial dose of MMI (or carbamizole) is 2.5 mg every 8 or 12 hours, depending on H+ severity and TH concentration, increasing to 5 mg in very severe cases or in cases of thyroid carcinoma. The initial dose in dogs is 5–20 mg every 12 hours (10–20 mg in cases of thyroid carcinoma). Propranolol is indicated for concurrent administration with MMI, at a dose of 0.2–1 mg/kg in dogs and 2.5 mg in cats (up to a maximum of 6.25 mg, depending on the animal's response). In both species it is administered every 12 hours, or every 8 hours if tachycardia and blood pressure are uncontrolled. Body weight should be measured every 15 days (it should stabilise and begin to recover) and TH levels should be re-evaluated after 30–45 days (Fig. 6). Once these are within reference ranges, definitive treatment can be instituted:

- Ablative dose of ^{131}I (first choice in cases of bilateral goitre and ectopic thyroid).
- Thyroid gland surgery, either partial (in cases of unilateral affectation, adenoma, or carcinoma) or total (does not respond to MMI or carbimazole and an ablative dose of ^{131}I is unavailable or contraindicated).
- Continue with a minimum dose of MMI to maintain euthyroid state (if an ablative dose of ^{131}I is unavailable or contraindicated). In the case of prolonged treatment, the MMI dose can be reduced to the lowest dose necessary to maintain a euthyroid state, monitoring TH and renal function and performing a complete blood count every 3 months (in cases of leukopenia MMI treatment should be discontinued).

REFERENCES

Cushing's syndrome

1. Galac S, Reusch CE, Kooistra HS et al. Adrenals. In: Rijnberk A, Kooistra HS, editors. *Clinical endocrinology of dogs and cats*. 2nd edition. Hannover (Germany): Schlütersche; 2010.
2. Quereda V, Malumbres M. Cell cycle control of pituitary development and disease. J Mol Endocrinol. 2009; 42: 75–86.
3. de Bruin C, Hanson JM, Meij BP et al. Expression and functional analysis of dopamine receptor subtype 2 and somatostatin receptor subtypes in canine Cushing's disease. *Endocrinol*. 2008; 149: 4357–4366.
4. Tanaka S. Comparative aspects of intracellular proteolytic processing of peptide hormone precursors: studies of proopiomelanocortin processing. *Zoolog Sci*. 2003; 20: 1183–1198.
5. Hereñú C, Rimoldi O, Becú-Villalobos D et al. Restorative effect of insulin-like growth factor-I gene therapy in the hypothalamus of senile rats with dopaminergic dysfunction. *Gene Ther*. 2006; 13: 1–9.
6. Pessina P, Fernández-Foren A, Cueto E et al. 2009. Cortisol secretion after adrenocorticotrophin (ACTH) and dexamethasone tests in healthy female and male dogs. *Acta Vet Scand*. 2009; 51: 33–37.
7. Bornstein SR, Engeland WC, Ehrhart-Bornstein M et al. Dissociation of ACTH and glucocorticoids. *Trends Endocrinol Metab*. 2008; 19: 175–180.
8. Kooistra HS, Galac S. Recent advances in the diagnosis of Cushing's syndrome in dogs. *Vet Clin North Am Small Anim Pract*. 2010; 40: 259–267.
9. Churcher RK. Hepatic carcinoid, hypercortisolism and hypokalaemia in a dog. *Aust Vet J*. 1999; 77: 641–645.
10. Galac S, Kooistra HS, Voorhout G et al. Hyperadrenocorticism in a dog due to ectopic secretion of adrenocorticotropic hormone. *Domest Anim Endocrinol*. 2005; 28:338–348.
11. Castillo VA, Pessina PP, Garcia JD et al. Ectopic ACTH syndrome in a dog with a mesenteric neuroendocrine tumour: a case report. *Vet Medicina*. 2014; 59: 352–358.

12. Galac S, Kars VJ, Voorhout G et al. ACTH-independent hyperadrenocorticism due to food-dependent hypercortisolemia in a dog: a case report. *Vet J.* 2008; 177: 141–143.
13. Galac S, Kars VJ, Klarenbeek S et al. Expression of receptors for luteinizing hormone, gastric-inhibitory polypeptide, and vasopressin in normal adrenal glands and cortisol-secreting adrenocortical tumors in dogs. *Domest Anim Endocrinol.* 2010; 39: 63–75.
14. Schoemaker NJ, van der Hage MH, Flik G et al. Morphology of the pituitary gland in ferrets (Mustela putorius furo) with hyperadrenocorticism. *J Comp Pathol.* 2004; 130: 255–265.
15. Gallelli MF, Cabrera Blatter MF, Castillo V. A comparative study by age and gender of the pituitary adenoma and ACTH and α-MSH secretion in dogs with pituitary-dependent hyperadrenocorticism. *Res Vet Sci.* 2010; 88: 33–40.
16. Castillo V, Wolberg A, Ghersevich MC. 2006. Cushing subagudo en el perro. *Redvet.* http://www.veterinaria.org, 7 (11): 111106//110626.
17. Willeberg P, Priester WA. Epidemiological aspects of clinical hyperadrenocorticism in dogs (canine Cushing's syndrome). *J Am Anim Hosp Assoc.* 1982; 18: 717–724.
18. Behrend EN, Kooistra HS, Nelson R et al. Diagnosis of spontaneous canine hyperadrenocorticism: 2012. ACVIM consensus statement (small animal). *J Vet Intern Med.* 2013; 27: 1292–1304.
19. Galac S, Kooistra HS, Teske E et al. Urinary corticoid/creatinine ratios in the differentiation between pituitary-dependent hyperadrenocorticism and hyperadrenocorticism due to adrenocortical tumour in the dog. Vet Q. 1997; 19: 17–20.
20. Mogicato G, Layssol-Lamour C, Conchou F et al. Ultrasonographic evaluation of the adrenal glands in healthy dogs: repeatability, reproducibility, observer-dependent variability, and the effect of bodyweight, age and sex. *Vet Rec.* 2011; 168: 130.
21. Ródenas S, Pumarola M, Gaitero L et al. Magnetic resonance imaging findings in 40 dogs with histologically confirmed intracranial tumours. *Vet J.* 2011; 187: 85–91.
22. Fleseriu M. Recent advances in the medical treatment of Cushing's disease. *Reports.* 2014; 6: 18 (doi: 10.12703/P6-18).
23. Hanson JM, Teske E, Voorhout G et al. Prognostic factors for outcome after transsphenoidal hypophysectomy in dogs with pituitary-dependent hyperadrenocorticism. *J Neurosurg.* 2007; 107: 830–840.
24. Reine N. Medical management of pituitary-dependent hyperadrenocorticism: mitotane versus trilostane. *Clin Tech Small Anim Pract.* 2007; 22: 18–25.
25. Feldman EC. Evaluation of twice-daily lower-dose trilostane treatment administered orally in dogs with naturally occurring hyperadrenocorticism. *J Am Vet Med Assoc.* 2011; 238: 1441–1451.
26. Ortemberg L, Loiza M, Martiarena B et al. Retinoic acid as a therapy for Cushing's disease in dogs: evaluation of liver enzymes during treatment. *Slov Vet Res.* 2007; 44: 73–81.
27. Teshima T, Hara Y, Takekoshi S et al. Trilostane-induced inhibition of cortisol secretion results in reduced negative feedback at the hypothalamic–pituitary axis. *Domest Anim Endocrinol.* 2009; 36: 32–44
28. Castillo VA, Gallelli MF. Corticotroph adenoma in the dog: pathogenesis and new therapeutic possibilities. *Res Vet Sci.* 2010; 88: 26–32.
29. Castillo V, Gómez N, Lalia J et al. Cushing's disease in dogs: cabergoline treatment. Res Vet Sci. 2008; 85: 26-34.
30. Castillo V, Giacomini D, Páez-Pereda M et al. Retinoic acid as a novel medical therapy for Cushing's disease in dogs. *Endocrinology.* 2006; 147: 4438-4444.
31. Castillo V, Theodoropoulou M, Stalla J et al. Effect of SOM230 (pasireotide) on corticotropic cells: action in dogs with Cushing's disease. *Neuroendocrinology.* 2011; 94: 124–136.
32. Ronchi CL, Kroiss M, Sbiera S et al. Current and evolving treatment options in adrenocortical carcinoma: where do we stand and where do we want to go? *Eur J Endocrinol.* 2014; 171: R1-R11.

Adrenal insufficiency

1. Beuschlein F. Regulation of aldosterone secretion: from physiology to disease. *Eur J Endocrinol.* 2013; 168: R85-R93.
2. Van Lanen K, Sande A. Canine hypoadrenocorticism: pathogenesis, diagnosis, and treatment. *Top Companion Anim Med.* 2014; 29: 88–95.
3. Thompson AL, Scott-Moncrieff JC, Anderson JD. Comparison of classic hypoadrenocorticism with glucocorticoid-deficient hypoadrenocorticism in dogs: 46 cases (1985-2005). *J Am Vet Med Assoc.* 2007; 230: 1190-1194.
4. Schmeitzel LP, Lothrop CD, Rosenkrantz WS. Congenital adrenal hyperplasia-like syndrome. In: Bonagura, JD. ed. *Kirk's Current Veterinary Therapy XII*. Philadelphia: WB Saunders. 1995: 600-4.
5. Frank LA, Hnilica KA, Rohrbach BW et al. Retrospective evaluation of sex hormones and steroid hormone intermediates in dogs with alopecia. *Vet Dermatol.* 2003; 14: 91-97.
6. Tyler J, Lathan P. Canine hypoadrenocorticism: pathogenesis and clinical features. *Comp Cont Educ Pract.* 2005; 27: 110-120.
7. Seth M, Drobatz KJ, Church DB et al. White blood cell count and the sodium to potassium ratio to screen for hypoadrenocorticism in dogs. *J Vet Intern Med.* 2011; 25: 1351-1356.
8. Wenzel K, Samal R, Hammer E et al. Pathophysiological aldosterone levels modify the secretory activity of cardiac progenitor cells. *Mol Cell Endocrinol.* 2017; 439: 16-25.

Hypothyroidism

1. Kaptein EM, Hays MT, Ferguson DC. Thyroid hormone metabolism. A comparative evaluation. *Vet Clin North Am Small Anim Pract.* 1994; 24: 431–466.
2. Daminet S, Ferguson DC. Influence of drugs on thyroid function in dogs. *J Vet Intern Med.* 2003; 17: 463–472
3. Larsen PR, Silva JE, Kaplan MM. Relationships between circulating and intracellular thyroid hormones: Physiological and clinical implications. *Endocr Rev.* 1981; 2 : 87–102.
4. Kaptein EM, Moore GE, Ferguson DC et al. Thyroxine and triiodothyronine distribution and metabolism in thyroxine-replaced athyreotic dogs and normal humans. *Am J Physiol.* 1993; 264: E90–E100.
5. Patel P, Landers K, Li H et al. Delivery of maternal thyroid hormones to the fetus. *Trends Endocrinol Metab.* 2011; 22: 164–170.
6. Castillo V. Canine hypothyroidism. *Vet Focus: Endocrine diseases.* 2011; 21: 2–8.
7. Graham PA, Refsal KR, Nachreiner RF. Etiopathologic findings of canine hypothyroidism. *Vet Clin North Am Small Anim Pract.* 2007; 37: 617-631.
8. Ferm K, Björnerfeldt S, Karlsson A *et al.* Prevalence of diagnostic characteristics indicating canine autoimmune lymphocytic thyroiditis in giant Schnauzer and Hovawart dogs. *J Small Anim Pract.* 2009; 50: 176–179.
9. Cooper DS, Biondi B. Subclinical thyroid disease. *Lancet.* 2012; 379:1142–1154.
10. Castillo V, Rodriguez MS, Lallia J. TSH response to TRH stimulation test on dogs. Diagnostic importance on subclinic thyroid disease (hypothyroidism and euthyroid autoimmune thyroiditis). *Revista Científica.* 2001; 11: 35–40.
11. Gonzalez E, Quadri SK. Effects of aging on the pituitary-thyroid axis in the dog. *Exp Gerontol.* 1988; 23: 151–160.
12. Ramírez Benavides GF, Osorio JR. Free tetraiodothyronine (FT4) serum levels by electrochemiluminescence method in canines. *Revista Científica.* 2009; 9: 238–241.
13. Bojanic K, Acke E, Jones BR. Congenital hypothyroidism of dogs and cats: a review. *NZ Vet J.* 2011; 59: 115–122.
14. Fyfe JC, Kampschmidt K, Dang V et al. 2003. Congenital hypothyroidism with goiter in toy fox terriers. *J Vet Intern Med.* 2003; 17: 50–57.
15. Dodgson SE, Day R, Fyfe JC. Congenital hypothyroidism with goiter in Tenterfield terriers. *J Vet Intern Med.* 2012; 26:1350–1357.
16. Mazrier H, French A, Ellinwood NM et al. Goitrous congenital hypothyroidism caused by thyroid peroxidase deficiency in a family of domestic shorthair cats. *J Vet Intern Med.* 2003; 17: 395–396.
17. Jones BR, Gruffydd-Jones TJ, Sparkes AH et al. Preliminary studies on congenital hypothyroidism in a family of Abyssinian cats. *Vet Rec.* 1992; 131: 145–148.
18. Sinha RA, Singh BK, Yen PM. Thyroid hormone regulation of hepatic lipid and carbohydrate metabolism. *Trends Endocrinol Metab.* 2014; 25: 538–545.
19. Kasamatsu M, Kawaichi R, Tsunokawa M et al. Comparison of serum lipid compositions, lipid peroxide, α-tocopherol and lipoproteins in captive marine mammals (bottlenose dolphins, spotted seals and West Indian manatees) and terrestrial mammals. *Res Vet Sci.* 2009; 86: 216–222.

20. Boretti FS, Reusch CE. Endogenous TSH in the diagnosis of hypothyroidism in dogs. *Schweiz Arch Tierheilkd*. 2004; 146: 183–188.
21. Castillo VA, Lalia JC, Junco M et al. Changes in thyroid function in puppies fed a high iodine commercial diet. *Vet J*. 2001; 161: 80–84.
22. Taeymans O, Penninck DG, Peters RM. Comparison between clinical, ultrasound, CT, MRI, and pathology findings in dogs presented for suspected thyroid carcinoma. *Vet Radiol Ultrasound*. 2013; 54: 61–70.
23. Le Traon G, Brennan SF, Burgaud S et al. Clinical evaluation of a novel liquid formulation of L-thyroxine for once daily treatment of dogs with hypothyroidism. *J Vet Internal Med*. 2009; 23: 43–49.
24. Iemura R, Toyota M, Micallef MJ. Effects of type of diet on pharmacokinetics of levothyroxine sodium oral solution. *Res Vet Sci*. 2013; 94: 695–697.
25. Liu YY, Brent GA. Thyroid hormone crosstalk with nuclear receptor signaling in metabolic regulation. *Trends Endocrinol Metab*. 2010; 21: 166–173.
26. Xenoulis PG, Steiner JM. Lipid metabolism and hyperlipidemia in dogs. *Vet J*. 2010; 183: 12–21.
27. Bhumika S, Darras VM. Role of thyroid hormones in different aspects of nervous system regeneration in vertebrates. *Gen Comp Endocrinol*. 2014; 203: 86–94.
28. Ahmed OM, El-Gareib AW, El-Bakry AM et al. Thyroid hormones states and brain development interactions. *Int. J. Dev Neurosci*. 2008; 26: 147-209.
29. Biondi B. Heart failure and thyroid dysfunction. *Eur J Endocrinol*. 2012; 167: 609–618.
30. Laurberg P, Cerqueira C, Ovesen L et al. Iodine intake as a determinant of thyroid disorders in populations. *Best Pract Res Clin Endocrinol Metab*. 2010; 24: 13–27.
31. Castillo V, Gambaro G, Sinatra V. Toxoplasmosis as a cause of subacute thyroiditis in dogs. *REDVET* 7 (3). 2006; http://www.veterinaria.org/revistas/redvet/n030306.html

Hyperthyroidism

1. Cooper DS, Biondi B. Subclinical thyroid disease. *Lancet*. 2012; 379: 1142–1154.
2. Mooney CT, Peterson ME. Feline hyperthyroidism. In: Mooney CT, Peterson ME, eds. *BSAVA Manual of Canine and Feline Endocrinology* (4th ed), Quedgeley, Gloucester: British Small Animal Veterinary Association; 2012: 199–203.
3. Syme HM. Cardiovascular and renal manifestations of hyperthyroidism. *Vet Clin North Am Small Anim Pract*. 2007; 37: 723–743.
4. Feldman EC, Nelson RW. Canine thyroid tumors and hyperthyroidism. In: Feldman EC, Nelson RW (eds.) *Canine and feline endocrinology and reproduction* (3rd ed). WB Saunders, St. Louis (MO); 2004: 219–249.
5. Barber LG. Thyroid tumors in dogs and cats. *Vet Clin North Am Small Anim Pract*. 2007; 37: 756-773.
6. Castillo V, Pessina P, Hall P et al. Post-surgical treatment of thyroid carcinoma in dogs with retinoic acid 9 cis improves patient outcome. *Open Vet J*. 2016; 6: 6–14.
7. Scott-Moncrieff JC. Thyroid disorders in the geriatric veterinary patient. *Vet Clin North Am Small Anim Pract*. 2012; 42: 707–725.
8. Graves TK, Peterson ME. Diagnosis of occult hyperthyroidism in cats. *Problems in veterinary medicine*. Philadelphia, PA, Lippincott. 1990: 683–692.
9. Peterson ME. 2001. Diagnostic of occult hyperthyroidism. In: *Consultations in Feline Internal Medicine* (4th ed). 2001; 145-150. Ed August.JR, Philadelphia, PA, USA: WB Saunders.
10. Wakeling J, Smith K, Scase T et al. Subclinical hyperthyroidism in cats: a spontaneous model of subclinical toxic nodular goiter in humans? *Thyroid*. 2007; 17: 1201–1209.
11. Peterson ME, Ward CR. Etiopathologic findings of hyperthyroidism in cats. *Vet Clin North Am Small Anim Pract*. 2007; 37: 633–645.
12. Peterson ME. Hyperthyroidism in cats: what's causing this epidemic of thyroid disease and can we prevent it? *J Feline Med Surg*. 2012; 14: 804–818.
13. Peterson ME. Feline hyperthyroidism: an animal model for toxic nodular goiter. *J Endocrinol*. 2014; 223: 197–1114.
14. Holzapfel HP, Bergner B, Wonerow P et al. Expression of Gαs proteins and TSH receptor signalling in hyperfunctioning thyroid nodules with TSH receptor mutations. *Eur J Endocrinol*. 2002; 147: 109–116.
15. Hammer KB, Holt DE, Ward CR. Altered expression of G proteins in thyroid gland adenomas obtained from hyperthyroid cats. *Am J Vet Res*. 2000; 61: 874–879.
16. Kopp P. The TSH receptor and its role in thyroid disease. *Cell Mol Life Sci*. 2001; 58: 1301–1322.
17. Pearce SH, Foster DJ, Imrie H et al. Mutational analysis of the thyrotropin receptor gene in sporadic and familial feline thyrotoxicosis. *Thyroid*. 1997; 7: 923–927.
18. Peeters ME, Timmermans-Sprang EP, Mol JA. Feline thyroid adenomas are in part associated with mutations in the G_{sa} gene and not with polymorphisms found in the thyrotropin receptor. *Thyroid*. 2002; 12: 571–575.
19. Watson SG, Radford AD, Kipar A et al. Somatic mutations of the thyroid-stimulating hormone receptor gene in feline hyperthyroidism: parallels with human hyperthyroidism. *J Endocrinol*. 2005; 186: 523–537.
20. Nguyen LQ, Arseven OK, Gerber H et al. Cloning of the cat TSH receptor and evidence against an autoimmune etiology of feline hyperthyroidism. *Endocrinology*. 2002; 143: 395–402.
21. Edinboro CH, Scott-Moncrieff JC, Glickman LT. Feline hyperthyroidism: potential relationship with iodine supplement requirements of commercial cat foods. *J Feline Med Surg*. 2010; 12: 672–679.
22. van der Kooij M, Becvarova I, Meyer HP et al. Effects of an iodine-restricted food on client-owned cats with hyperthyroidism. *J Feline Med Surg*. 2013; 14: 491–498.
23. Hui TY, Bruyette DS, Moore GE et al. Effect of feeding an iodine-restricted diet in cats with spontaneous hyperthyroidism. *J Vet Intern Med*. 2015; 29: 1063–1068.
24. Hibbert A, Gruffydd-Jones T, Barrett EL et al. Feline thyroid carcinoma: diagnosis and response to high-dose radioactive iodine treatment. *J Feline Med Surg*. 2009; 11: 116–124.
25. Peterson ME, Broome MR. Thyroid scintigraphy findings in 2,096 cats with hyperthyroidism. *Vet Radiol Ultrasound*. 2015; 56: 84–95.
26. Wakeling J, Elliott J, Syme H. Evaluation of predictors for the diagnosis of hyperthyroidism in cats. *J Vet Intern Med*. 2011; 25: 1057–1065.
27. Peterson ME. Diagnostic tests for hyperthyroidism in cats. *Clin Tech Small Anim Pract*. 2006; 21: 2–9.
28. Peterson ME, Melian C, Nichols R. Measurement of serum concentrations of free thyroxine, total thyroxine, and total triiodothyronine in cats with hyperthyroidism and cats with nonthyroidal disease. *J Am Vet Med Assoc*. 2001; 218: 529–536.
29. Peterson ME, Graves TK, Gamble DA. Triiodothyronine (T3) suppression test. An aid in the diagnosis of mild hyperthyroidism in cats. *J Vet Intern Med*. 1990; 4: 233–238.
30. Castillo V, Gambaro G, Sinatra V. Toxoplasmosis as a cause of subacute thyroiditis in dogs. *REDVET* 7 (3). 2006; http://www.veterinaria.org/revistas/redvet/n030306.html.
31. Ferguson DC. Testing for hypothyroidism in dogs. *Vet Clin North Am Small Anim Pract*. 2007; 37: 647–669.
32. Daniel GB, Neelis DA. Thyroid scintigraphy in veterinary medicine. *Semin Nucl Med*. 2014; 44: 24–34.
33. Volckaert V, Vandermeulen E, Duchateau L et al. Inter- and intraobserver variability of (semi-)quantitative parameters commonly used in feline thyroid scintigraphy. *Res Vet Sci*. 2016; 105: 87–91.
34. Trepanier L, Hoffman SB, Kroll M et al. Efficacy and safety of once versus twice daily administration of methimazole in cats with hyperthyroidism. *J Am Vet Med Assoc*. 2003; 222: 954–958.
35. Daminet S, Kooistra HS, Fracassi F et al. Best practice for the pharmacological management of hyperthyroid cats with antithyroid drugs. *J Small Anim Pract*. 2014; 55: 4–13.
36. Fritsch DA, Allen TA, Dodd DE et al. A restricted iodine food reduces circulating thyroxine concentrations in cats with hyperthyroidism. *Int J Appl Res Vet Med*. 2014; 12: 24–32.
37. Naan EC, Kirpensteijn J, Kooistra HS et al. Results of thyroidectomy in 101 cats with hyperthyroidism. *Vet Surg*. 2006; 35: 287–293.